Wound Care Management

Third Edition

Wound Care Management

A Person-Centred Approach

Edited by
Sebastian Probst DClinPrac, MNS, RN
Professor of Tissue Viability and Wound Care, School of Health Sciences
HES-SO, University of Applied Sciences and Arts Western Switzerland
Geneva, Switzerland

Foreword writer
Sue Bale OBE, PhD, BA, RGN, NDN, RHV, Dip N
Professor, Director of Research & Development in Aneurin Bevan Health Board
Wales, UK

ELSEVIER

Edinburgh   London   New York   Oxford   Philadelphia   St Louis   Sydney   2021

First edition 1997
Second edition 2006
Third edition 2021

Notices

Practitioners and researchers must always rely on their own experience and knowledge in evaluating and using any information, methods, compounds or experiments described herein. Because of rapid advances in the medical sciences, in particular, independent verification of diagnoses and drug dosages should be made. To the fullest extent of the law, no responsibility is assumed by Elsevier, authors, editors or contributors for any injury and/or damage to persons or property as a matter of products liability, negligence or otherwise, or from any use or operation of any methods, products, instructions, or ideas contained in the material herein.

ISBN: 978-0-7020-7981-8

Content Strategist: Serena Castelnovo, Poppy Garraway Smith
Content Development Specialist: Fiona Conn
Project Manager: Julie Taylor
Design: Bridget Hoette
Illustration Manager: Nararyanan Ramakrishnan
Marketing Manager: Kristen Oyirifi

Printed in China

Last digit is the print number: 9 8 7 6 5 4 3 2 1

Contents

Foreword

In modern healthcare today, wound management is accepted as a legitimate and fundamental aspect of patient care. This was not always the case and it was only in the last century that we saw the evolution of wound specialists, wound care societies, research and innovation and wound education. For many patients these developments have transformed their care as they can access organised, evidence-based wound healing services, producing improvements in outcomes and quality of life.

Progress continues, and health professionals are increasingly recognising the importance of putting the patient at the centre of all they do. Across Europe and further afield, health policy supports this view that working in partnership with patients to design and deliver healthcare is critical to successful patient outcomes. This includes collecting patient-reported outcome measures and patient-reported experience measures, which inform the development of services. The underpinning principle in the third edition of *Wound Care Nursing: A Person-centred Approach* is to place the patient at the centre of care.

Nurses and other health professionals encounter patients with wounds on an almost daily basis. As nurses usually spend more time with patients than any other health professional, they plan and provide the vast majority of wound care. However, many textbooks on wound care that nurses access adopt a medical model of disease types and wound aetiologies. Whilst these approaches are useful, they miss the unique aspects of nursing. This book uses an holistic approach to wound care by deploying nursing models to illustrate how patients' care across the life cycle can planned, delivered and evaluated.

The editor, Sebastian Probst, has brought together an impressive selection of experts who share their expertise in a highly readable text. Readers are given aetiology, epidemiology, assessment, planning and evaluation throughout the lifecycle. Every part of patients' lifecycle is illustrated by case studies, which are based on real patient stories. This method of teaching reflects experiential learning, by far the most effective way to learn and remember what we've learnt.

The new edition will be useful to specialist and generalist nurses and other health professionals caring for patients with wounds in all healthcare settings across Europe and beyond. It should be widely available as it will help practitioners apply the theory they learn to practice.

The burden of wound care in terms of patient morbidity and mortality is often higher than it needs to be. Combined with the devastating personal costs to patients and high financial costs, these are very good reasons to prevent as many wounds as possible and to improve wound care ensuring wounds heal quickly and effectively. I highly recommend this book to all those seeking to improve patient care.

Professor Sue Bale OBE, PhD, BA, RGN, NDN, RHV, DipN

Preface and Acknowledgement

The aim of this book is to support nurses in clinical practice when taking care of patients with a wound. The book is designed to picture the circle of life with its different wounds and their problems. This updated version includes two new chapters: a chapter about incontinence-associated dermatitis and one about palliative wound care. Each chapter starts with key issues, followed by an evidence-based discussion of the topic with case studies and concludes with multiple-choice questions for review.

I would like to thank Sue and Vanessa, the editors of the first and second editions of this book, for their confidence shown in me for editing their book. Additionally, I would like to thank all the authors for their valuable contributions.

SP

List of Contributors

The editor would like to acknowledge and offer grateful thanks for the input of all previous editions' contributors, without whom this new edition would not have been possible.

Dimitri Beeckman, BSc, MSc, PhD
Professor, University Centre for Nursing and Midwifery, Ghent University, Ghent, Belgium; Professor, School of Nursing and Midwifery, Royal College for Surgeons in Ireland, Dublin, Ireland; Professor, School of Health Sciences, Örebro University, Örebro, Sweden

Paul Bobbink, MSN
Lecturer, Geneva School of Health Sciences, HES-SO University of Applied Sciences and Arts Western Switzerland, Geneva, Switzerland

Georgina Gethin, PhD, MSc Clinical Research, PG Dip Wound Healing, RGN, Dip Anatomy, Dip Applied Physiology, FFNM RCSI
Senior Lecturer, Head of School, Nursing and Midwifery, NUI Galway, Galway, Ireland; Director, Alliance for Research and Innovation in Wounds, NUI Galway, Galway, Ireland; Adjunct Associate Professor, Nursing and Midwifery, Monash University, Australia

Sinéad Mary Hahessy, BA, MA (SocSc)
Lecturer/Programme Director for the Postgraduate Diploma in Nursing, National University of Ireland Galway (NUIG), Galway, Ireland

Samantha Holloway, MSc
Reader/Programme Director, Centre for Medical Education, Cardiff University Heath Park Campus, Cardiff, UK

Andrea Pokorná, MSc, PhD
Professor, Department of Nursing and Midwifery, Institute of Biostatistic and Analyses, Masaryk University, Czech Republic

Sebastian Probst, DClinPrac, MSN, RN
Professor of Tissue Viability and Wound Care, Geneva School of Health Sciences, HES-SO University of Applied Sciences and Arts Western Switzerland, Geneva, Switzerland

Anna-Barbara Schlüer, PhD, MScN
Doctor, Pediatric Skin Center – Skin and Wound Management, Children's University Hospital, Zurich, Switzerland

Brecht Serraes, MSc, RN
PhD student, Skin Integrity Research Group (SKINT), University Centre for Nursing and Midwifery, Department of Public Health and Primary Care, Ghent University, Ghent, Belgium; Process Manager, Nursing Department, AZ Nikolaas General Hospital, Sint-Niklaas, Belgium

ASSESSMENT AND PLANNING

Chapter 1

Assessing the Normal and Abnormal

Georgina Gethin

Highlights

- Wound healing is a complex, non-linear, staged process that is influenced at each stage by intrinsic and extrinsic factors that can delay or promote healing
- The nurse assessing the wound should have a comprehensive knowledge of the healing process and of methods to assess the patient and their wound
- Signs of infection in chronic wounds are less obvious than in acute wounds and include but are not limited to: increasing wound pain, increasing wound size, malodour and friable granulation tissue
- Supporting and informing patients to help them achieve a well-balanced diet is vital to wound healing and to patient well-being

Key Issues

This chapter introduces the reader to the factors that need to be considered in order to perform a full assessment. The following areas are covered:
- Assessment of the individual
  - Normal stages of healing
  - Abnormalities of healing
  - Wound healing by primary and secondary intention
- Factors that affect healing
  - Intrinsic
  - Extrinsic
- Assessment of the wound
  - Sutured/granulating
  - Shape and size
  - Recognition of infection
- Assessment of the environment
  - Hospital or community based

Introduction

Planning individualized patient care commences with a comprehensive and holistic assessment (Fig. 1.1). Achieving this requires knowledge of the aetiology of wounds, of the healing process and of the intrinsic and extrinsic factors that can delay or promote wound healing. This chapter will focus on those factors which should be considered in completing the assessment.

Assessment of the Individual

Assessment of the overall health of the individual will highlight factors that may impair the normal healing process. Before an understanding of these factors can be appreciated it is essential that the nurse has a sound knowledge of the healing process.

A multiplicity of wound assessment tools exist and it is beyond the scope of this chapter to review these, but it is worth noting that the validity and reliability of many of the methods used to assess the wound bed is either very low or in some cases non-existent.[1] A recently published tool (Triangle) encompasses wound factors, including the wound bed, wound edge and periwound area, together with patient factors, including clinical history and clinical examination, and provides an option that nurses may wish to adapt to their setting.[2]

NORMAL WOUND HEALING

Wound healing is a complex chain of events that can be divided into its four constituent phases – haemostasis, inflammation, proliferation and maturation (Fig. 1.2) – all of which overlap at some point and do not all occur in a sequential manner.

Haemostasis

Following cutaneous injury to blood vessels and endothelial cells, blood extravasation into the wound

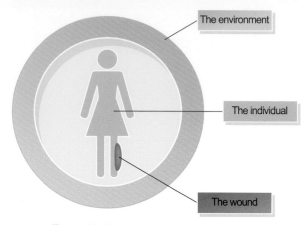

Fig. 1.1 A holistic approach to wound assessment.

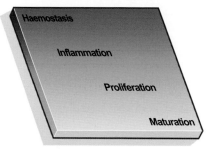

Fig. 1.2 The wound healing process. Although for convenience the wound healing process is considered here in four phases, it is important to remember that healing is a dynamic, ongoing process. It begins at day 0 with initial wounding but can continue for several years.

defect exposes the blood to various components of the extracellular matrix (ECM).[3] Platelets aggregate and degranulate, resulting in clot formation and haemostasis. Haemostasis is the arrest of haemorrhage at the site of blood vessel damage and is essential as it preserves the integrity of the closed and high-pressure circulatory system to limit blood loss (Fig. 1.3). A fibrinous clot forms during coagulation. This acts as a preliminary matrix within the wound space into which cells can migrate. A short period of vasoconstriction occurs owing to the release of chemical mediators such as histamine, serotonin and adenosine triphosphate (ATP). Most of these mediators act as chemoattractants to circulating leucocytes, bringing them to the injured area.

Following initial vasoconstriction, the inflammatory process begins with the release of prostaglandins and activated complement proteins, causing widespread vasodilation and inflammation.[4]

Inflammatory Phase

As the fibrin clot is degraded, the capillaries dilate and become permeable, thus allowing plasma to leak into the surrounding tissue, producing inflammatory exudate.[5] This activates the complement system, composed of a series of interacting, soluble proteins found in serum and extracellular fluid that induce lysis and destruction of target cells, such as bacteria. Cytokines and some proteolytic fragments that are chemoattractive are also found in the wound space.[6] Their abundance and accumulation at the site of wounding initiate a massive influx of other cells.

The two main inflammatory cells are neutrophils and macrophages.[5] Neutrophils appear in a wound shortly after injury and reach their peak number within 24–48 hours. Their main function is to destroy bacteria by the process of phagocytosis. Neutrophils have a very short lifespan and their numbers reduce rapidly after 3 days in the absence of infection. Monocytes undergo a phenotypic change to become activated macrophages, which produce growth factors that start, accelerate or modify the healing process. Tissue macrophages, like neutrophils, destroy bacteria and debris through phagocytosis. The macrophage is also a rich source of biological regulators, including cytokines and growth factors, bioactive lipid products and proteolytic enzymes, which are also essential for the normal healing process.[7]

The formation of new blood vessels occurs with the release of angiogenic growth factors, which stimulate endothelium to divide and direct the growth of new blood vessels.[8]

Proliferative Phase

The macrophages next recruit a new type of cell, the fibroblast, which produces a network of collagen surrounding the neovasculature of the wound. Fibroblasts also produce proteoglycan, a glue-like ground substance which fills the tissue space, coating and binding fibres together to give them greater flexibility, and fibronectin, which forms the framework for tissue by holding collagen and cells together while attaching them to the ground substance.

The proliferation phase usually commences at about day 3 following injury and lasts for some weeks. This phase is characterized by the formation of granulation tissue in the wound space. This new tissue consists of a matrix of fibrin, fibronectin, collagens, proteoglycans and glycosaminoglycans and other

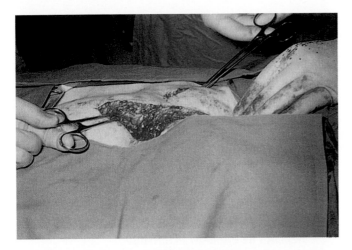

Fig. 1.3 Haemostasis.

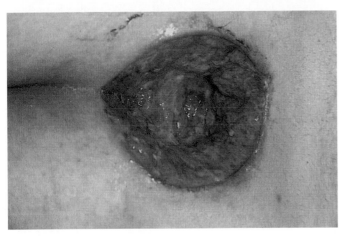

Fig. 1.4 Healthy granulation tissue on the wound bed of a pilonidal sinus excision. (Reproduced with kind permission from the *Journal of Wound Care*, London.)

glycoproteins.[9] Fibroblasts move into the wound space and proliferate; their function during wound healing is to synthesize and deposit extracellular proteins, producing growth factors and angiogenic factors that regulate cell proliferation and angiogenesis.[3,9,10]

Collagen is the most abundant protein in animal tissue and accounts for 70–80% of the dry weight of the dermis.[11] Mainly made by fibroblasts, there are at least 19 genetically distinct collagens currently identified. Collagen synthesis and degradation are finely balanced.[11] Elastin is a protein that provides wounds with elasticity and resilience.[11] Elastin fibres form coils that enable it to stretch and return to its former shape, much like metallic coils. Because of these properties, elastin helps to maintain tissue shape.

Wound exudate is initially produced in the inflammatory phase of healing,[12] although it continues to be produced throughout the healing phase until complete epithelialization has been achieved. Exudate has a high protein content and contains essential nutrients, as well as providing a moist environment.[12] These nutrients include plasma proteins, growth factors, proteolytic enzymes, glucose, lactic acid, white blood cells, macrophages, fibrin and platelets.[4,5,12]

Measuring and describing levels of exudate production for the purposes of evaluating progress towards healing and recording wound symptoms is largely a subjective process. Many scales have been developed to assess exudate but the validity and reliability of such scales has not been well assessed.[1]

The formation of new connective tissue (granulation tissue) is dependent on angiogenesis with the resultant formation of new blood vessels in the wound (Fig. 1.4). Initially the wound is hypoxic and lacking in nutrients, but as capillary loops are formed the environment becomes oxygenated.[8] Angiogenesis or formation of new vessels in the wound space is an integral and essential part of wound healing.[13] The major cell involved in angiogenesis is the vascular endothelial cell, which arises from the damaged end of vessels and capillaries. New vessels originate as capillaries, which sprout from existing small vessels at the wound edge. The endothelial cells from these vessels are detached from the vascular wall, degrade and penetrate (invade) the provisional matrix in the wound, thus forming a cone-shaped vascular bud or sprout. A sprout is then extended in length until it encounters another capillary and connects to form vascular loops and networks, allowing blood to circulate.

During proliferation, two other processes are taking place simultaneously – epithelialization and contraction. Epithelialization resurfaces the wound by regenerating epithelium. Where damage is extensive and involves deep dermal tissue loss, regeneration occurs from the wound margins. Where there is superficial skin loss, remnants of hair follicles will act as islands of regenerating epithelium. Migration across the wound surface continues until other epithelial cells are met. The migration then ceases – a complex process known as contact inhibition. Wound contraction decreases the size of the wound, due to the work of the myofibroblasts. Myofibroblasts under the influence of inflammatory mediators reduce the surface area of the wound before cellular proliferation takes place. The myofibroblast is a differentiated fibroblast containing actin and myosin fibrils.[7,14]

Once an open cavity has filled with new granulation tissue and epithelialization has occurred, the proliferative phase of healing stops.

Maturation Phase

The final stage of healing begins about 3 weeks after injury and is a process of remodelling of the collagen fibres laid down during the proliferation phase (Fig. 1.5).

During the maturation phase, type III collagen, a soft gelatinous collagen, is gradually replaced with stronger, more highly organized collagen. Differentiation of collagen is a dynamic process and although it commences during maturation, it may continue indefinitely.

Collagen breakdown and production is a finely balanced process which, if impaired, can result in delayed or inadequate healing. Once established, the amount of collagen bed does not alter, just the type and formation within the wound. Type III collagen is removed by collagenases and synthesis of type I collagen occurs, laid down in a more orderly network and fashioned along the lines of tension.

The process of remodelling continues with the fibroblasts migrating from the wound site and there is rationalization of the numerous blood vessels, resulting in shrinking, thinning and paling of the scar.

HEALING BY PRIMARY INTENTION

Healing by primary intention occurs following a clean surgical incision where the edges of the wound are closely approximated, thus eliminating dead space. There is minimal formation of granulation tissue and once the wound has healed, only a thin seam remains. All the above phases of wound healing occur but following the initial inflammatory response, wound contraction has a minor role and epithelium migrates over the suture line to restore tissue integrity.[15]

HEALING BY SECONDARY INTENTION

Healing by secondary intention (Fig. 1.6) occurs in wounds where there is a large tissue defect. The wound must heal by formation of granulation tissue and wound contraction, resulting in dense, fibrous scar tissue. These wounds take longer to heal because of the large amounts of granulation tissue required. The proliferative and maturation phases are longer than in wounds healing by primary intention.

HEALING BY THIRD INTENTION

Where the presence of infection or a foreign body is suspected, a wound may be left open to commence healing by granulation until the presenting problem has been resolved. The wound edges are then approximated and healing by primary intention can proceed.

ABNORMAL WOUND HEALING

Unfortunately, failure or delay in achieving adequate healing is common, especially for patients with chronic wounds. Abnormalities of wound healing are described below.

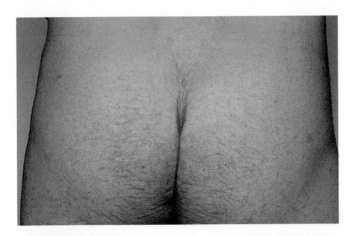

Fig. 1.5 A healed pilonidal sinus excision in the maturation phase.

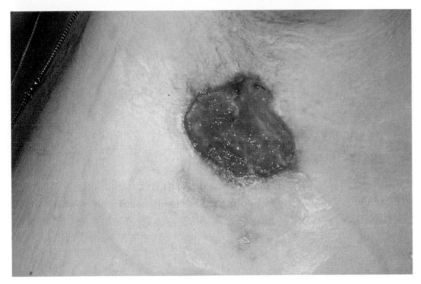

Fig. 1.6 An axillary wound healing by secondary intention.

Dehiscence

Dehiscence represents partial or complete separation of the outer layers of a sutured incision and occurs when the wound has failed to develop sufficient strength to withstand forces placed upon it. It is estimated to occur in 0.5–3.4% of abdominopelvic surgeries and carries a mortality rate of 40%.[16] In a study of 25,636 patients undergoing abdominopelvic surgery, 786 (2.97%) had wound dehiscence.[16] These patients were older, more commonly male and had a significantly higher body mass index (BMI) (*P* < .0001).[16] Of note, exposure to opioid agents in the 30 days following surgery was associated with dehiscence and remained so even when data were adjusted for infection (odds ratio (OR) 1.602, *P* < .001).[16]

The patient often presents with pyrexia and wound discharge of serosanguineous fluid. The risk is always increased by localized wound infection, haematoma formation or excessive tension placed on the wound by coughing. A major complication is the protrusion of an organ through the open wound, which can lead to peritonitis and/or septic shock.

Incisional Hernia

Incisional hernias are a major cause of morbidity (Fig. 1.7); they occur in up to 10% of abdominal wounds,[17] can develop months or even years following surgery and represent failure of part of the scar to develop sufficient strength. They occur more often in infected wounds and in obese patients. The risk factors include

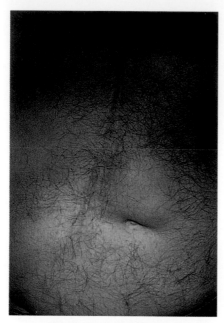

Fig. 1.7 An incisional hernia.

TABLE 1.1 Factors Adversely Affecting the Healing Process	
Intrinsic Factors	**Extrinsic Factors**
Age	Poor surgical technique
Disease processes/metabolic	Poor wound care
Psychological status	Malnutrition
Body image	Fluid balance
	Smoking
	Drug therapies
	Radiotherapy

hypoxia, immunosuppressant treatments, metabolic disorders, obesity, previous abdominal surgery, previous incisional hernia and wound dehiscence.[17]

Malignant Changes

Any long-standing ulcer may undergo malignant changes to form a squamous cell carcinoma. Although the precise mechanism is unknown, with such a rapid turnover of cells in any wound it is important that the practitioner should bear in mind the possibility of malignancy.

Any wound that has an unusual appearance or fails to heal over a long period should be investigated. Patients who have failed to heal or failed to show significant signs of healing over an expected period should be routinely biopsied to exclude malignancy.[18]

Factors Affecting Wound Healing

There are many factors, intrinsic and extrinsic, that can adversely affect the normal healing process and are listed in Table 1.1.

Assessment aims to identify these factors and, wherever possible, treat or prevent them. However, where this is not possible, factors known to affect healing should be documented and the possibility of delayed healing planned for.

INTRINSIC FACTORS

Age

During the ageing process the dermis of the skin gradually becomes thinner and the underlying structural support – collagen – diminishes at a rate of 1% per annum.[19] The dermis displays fewer fibroblasts, macrophages and mast cells, and has reduced vascularity and a loss of extracellular matrix (ECM) components, including collagen.[20] Besides the imbalance of collagen production and degradation, the quality of the remaining collagen is also altered, showing fewer rope-like bundles and a higher degree of disorganization.[20]

Skin loses elasticity as the fibroblasts responsible for elastin and collagen synthesis decline in number, elastic fibres thicken and the ability for elastic recoil is lost, resulting in creases and wrinkles. At the same time the amount of subcutaneous fat lessens, thus providing less of a cushion for underlying bone. Keratinocyte proliferation is reduced and the turnover time, i.e., the number of days for keratinocytes to migrate from the basal layer to the skin surface, is increased by 50%.[20] Additionally, natural moisture from sebum secretion reduces in old age as these sweat glands become smaller, leading to increased dryness of the skin. Tensile wound strength is often affected, owing to reduced collagen production and poor circulation associated with old age. Additional age-related changes are diminished sensation to light touch and pressure and a decreased capacity to produce vitamin D.[20] Overall, the ageing process adversely affects skin quality, causing dry, thin inelastic skin that is susceptible to damage.

Disease

A whole range of disease processes that adversely affect metabolism are also likely to delay or prevent wound healing:

- Anaemia
- Arteriosclerosis
- Cancer
- Cardiovascular disorders
- Diabetes
- Immune disorders
- Inflammatory diseases
- Jaundice, liver failure
- Rheumatoid arthritis
- Uraemia.

In many groups of patients, particularly those with venous leg ulceration, multimorbidity is common.[21]

Psychological Factors

There is a close association between the psychological and physical well-being of individuals. Stress and anxiety in particular can affect the immune system. Chronic stress increases cortisol release, which has an anti-inflammatory effect. This disrupts the normal functioning of immune cells required for the inflammatory phase of healing, thus delaying the process.[22] Stress adversely affects the normal barrier function of the skin.[23] Animal and human laboratory studies have also demonstrated the effects of stress on the sympathetic nervous system, where vasoactive substances (for example, catecholamines) impair perfusion to the wound bed.[24] Wound assessment plans should consider psychological factors that may delay healing and also address factors such as pain control, patient education and counselling. It is proposed that psychological interventions may improve healing outcomes in diabetic foot ulceration.[25]

Sleep disturbances are also linked with stress. Sleep encourages anabolism and, as wound healing includes anabolic processes, it has been suggested that healing is promoted by rest and sleep. Sleep is an important biological phenomenon for skin homeostasis and a shortage of sleep interferes with the barrier function of the skin.[23] Growth hormone is secreted during sleep, which in turn stimulates protein synthesis and fibroblast and endothelial cell proliferation.[26]

Body Image

Body image has been defined as an individual's perception of their own appearance, which may be quite different from their actual physical appearance.[27] Body image can be adversely altered or affected by a change in physical appearance such as traumatic injury, surgery or burns. Dramatic negative effects can occur, especially when disfiguring surgery has been performed such as mastectomy, stoma formation or the amputation of a limb. Altered body image is particularly distressing in malignant fungating wounds, where patients describe themselves as living in an 'unbounded body'.[28] The grieving process is associated with this negative alteration in body image[26]; common problems include a sense of loss, anxiety and withdrawal from social relationships.

EXTRINSIC FACTORS

Poor Surgical Technique

Specific situations which may impair healing include: inadequate closure of tissue layers, resulting in a dead space; inappropriate use of diathermy or drains; sutures inserted too tightly or too loosely; prolonged operating time and haematoma.[29] The most common of these problems is haematoma formation, caused by rough handling of tissues and by inappropriate use of diathermy or wound drains. This can lead to the presence of a dead space, encouraging wound infection as the haematoma is broken down. Complications from haematoma formation include: increased tension on the healing wound; excess fibrosis or scar tissue; and, most commonly, the medium provided for micro-organisms that increases the risk of infection and wound breakdown.

Poor Wound Care

Wound healing may be impeded by poor dressing technique or the inappropriate use of a dressing material or antiseptic solution. These problems can be avoided by the use of appropriate knowledge and skills in assessment and wound care.

Malnutrition

Adequate nutrition is a prerequisite to good wound healing. Malnutrition is a 'state of nutrition in which a deficiency, excess or imbalance of energy, protein

BOX 1.1 PATIENTS AT RISK OF HOSPITAL-INDUCED PROTEIN–ENERGY MALNUTRITION

1. Emergency admission
2. All age groups, but especially elderly individuals recently bereaved, socially isolated or with sensory or mental impairment
3. Malignancy, especially cancer of the gastrointestinal tract
4. Alimentary tract diseases
5. Dysphagia or anorexia

From Dickerson J. The problem of hospital-induced malnutrition. *Nurs Times.* 1995;91(4):44–45.

or other nutrients, including vitamins and minerals, causes measurable adverse effects on body function and clinical outcome'.[30] Malnutrition can result in delays in wound healing, causing weak, poor-quality scars. In reviewing the literature on malnutrition and healing, McLaren[31] and Stotts[32] describe two types of malnutrition that affect healing: protein–energy malnutrition (PEM) and nutrient deficiencies.

Protein–energy malnutrition

McLaren[31] defines PEM as a change in body composition and physiology that results from an absolute or relative deficiency of energy and protein, which affects between 19% and 50% of hospitalized patients. She attributes PEM to several factors, including a reduced intake of nutrients, reduced absorption and digestion of nutrients and increased metabolic use. McLaren[31] estimates that although 70% of these patients are malnourished prior to admission, the remaining 30% develop PEM during their hospital stay, as a complication.

Dickerson[33] identified a range of patients vulnerable to hospital-induced PEM (Box 1.1). McWhirter and Pennington[34] found that 200 out of 500 patients admitted to hospital were undernourished and just over 100 lost weight during their admission. Gray and Cooper[35] and the European Pressure Ulcer Advisory Panel (EPUAP)[36] recommend that nutritional screening tools should be used to identify patients at risk of being malnourished and that food record charts are also useful in ensuring that patients receive optimal care. Malnutrition can affect wound healing in several ways:

- poor wound healing, reduced tensile strength and increased wound dehiscence[32,33]
- increased susceptibility to infections[33]
- susceptibility to the development of pressure ulcers[33]
- poor-quality scarring.[37]

In older adults absorption and metabolism of nutrients are impaired because of the effects of ageing on the gastrointestinal tract and liver. With ageing, protein normally decreases, body water is reduced and there is a redistribution of fat stores as well as loss of bone density. Specific requirements for individual patients vary and depend on their body weight. The EPUAP nutrition guidelines[38] are based on a systematic review of the literature and recommend a minimum intake of 30–35 kcal per kg of body weight, with 1–1.5 g per kg per day protein and 1 mL per kcal per day of fluid intake. EPUAP[36] recommends that health professionals should consider the quality of the food being offered, along with removing physical or social barriers to its consumption. Although there is a lack of clear evidence from RCTs that nutritional interventions are beneficial for preventing and treating pressure ulcers, close monitoring of the patient's dietary intake is important for patients at risk of pressure ulceration as it is using a valid and reliable screening tool.[36] EPUAP also suggests that nutritional supplements be considered when it is not possible to enhance the patient's own consumption of food and fluids.

Common causes of malnutrition in the elderly include: decreased appetite; requiring assistance to eat; impaired cognition; poor positioning; frequent acute illness; medications that decrease appetite or increase nutrient loss; polypharmacy; decreased thirst response; monotony of diet; and intentional fluid restrictions because of fear of incontinence.[39] To improve nutrition, addressing impairments to dentition and swallowing, addressing physical or cognitive deficits and auditing of practice are all required in addition to appropriate assessment.

Trace element deficiency

Zinc is an essential cofactor for the enzymatic activity of 200 or more enzymes, including protein synthesis,[31,40] and zinc deficiency has long been known to impair wound healing.[35] Patients who are zinc deficient have reduced rates of epithelialization, decreased wound strength and reduced collagen synthesis.[37]

Copper is needed for the cross-linkage of collagen. Although rare, copper deficiency reduces the activity of an enzyme, lysyl oxidase, essential in collagen formation. Patients receiving long-term total parenteral nutrition and those with malabsorption syndrome are most at risk.[31]

Collagen synthesis relies on iron, as it is an essential cofactor for both lysyl and prolyl hydroxylase. In addition, anaemia may impair healing through reducing oxygen transportation.[31]

Vitamin C is essential for the synthesis of collagen. It functions as a cofactor in the hydroxylation of proline to hydroxyproline.[37] A deficiency in vitamin C results in impaired angiogenesis,[40] reduces tensile strength within wounds and increases capillary fragility.[31,35]

Vitamin A enhances the early inflammatory response, whilst stimulating fibroblast proliferation and increasing tensile strength.[40] It may also be linked to limiting wound infections as it is important in the normal human defence mechanism. It is also involved in the cross-linking of collagen and the proliferation of epithelial cells.[35] Supplements of vitamin A have been used to reverse the effects of corticosteroid treatments in patients to improve wound healing.[37]

Fluid Balance

In addition to an adequate intake of food, fluids are also required. Around 2000–2500 mL of fluid is required daily for efficient metabolism.

Smoking

Smoking has an adverse effect on the general health of individuals throughout their lives. There is a high correlation between smoking, lung cancer and cardiovascular diseases. Tobacco smoke contains nicotine and carbon monoxide. There are, however, differences between cigarette smoke and pipe or cigar smoke as far as nicotine is concerned; cigarettes are more harmful to health,[41] with more nicotine being absorbed and peripheral blood flow being depressed by at least 50% for more than an hour after smoking just one cigarette. In animal models nicotine has been shown to inhibit epithelialization.[42] A meta-analysis of the effects of smoking cessation on healing outcomes in surgical wounds has shown postoperative complications occur significantly less often in non-smokers compared to smokers.[43] Table 1.2 shows the

TABLE 1.2 The Main Influence of Nicotine and Carbon Monoxide on Peripheral Tissue in Relation to Wound Healing

Tissue	Nicotine	Carbon Monoxide	Total Effect
Skin	Contraction	Dilation	Contraction
Muscles	Dilation		Dilation
Oxygen supply	Reduced blood flow	Reduced oxygen transport	Reduced oxygen tension in tissue
Platelets	Increased aggregation	Increased aggregation	Formation of thrombi
Fibrin	Increased plasma concentration		No proven effect

Reproduced with permission from Siana JE, Frankjld S, Gottrup F. The effect of smoking on tissue function. *J Wound Care*. 1992;1(2):37–41.

effects of carbon monoxide and nicotine on blood vessels and blood components in relation to wound healing. Cessation of smoking 4 weeks prior to surgery has been shown to reduce surgical site infections.[43] In diabetic foot ulceration, smoking has an overall negative effect on wound healing, with average healing rates of 62% among smokers versus 71% in non-smokers (OR 0.70; 95% confidence interval (CI) 0.56–0.88).[44]

Drug Therapies

Drugs that interfere with cell proliferation can have a severe effect on wound healing. These are predominantly cytotoxic drugs, especially vincristine. However, the most commonly encountered drugs that adversely affect healing are the corticosteroids. When taken over a long period, they suppress fibroblast and collagen synthesis.

Radiotherapy

Depending on the dosage of radiotherapy used, wounds in the immediate vicinity of the treated area may fail to heal or heal slowly. Long-term weakness of the skin and other tissues can occur following radiotherapy.[45]

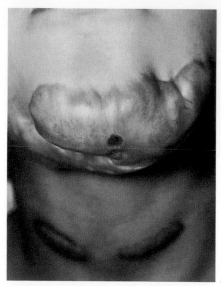

Fig. 1.8 Hypertrophic scarring (Reproduced with kind permission from Dr C. Lawrence, Wound Healing Research Unit, Cardiff.)

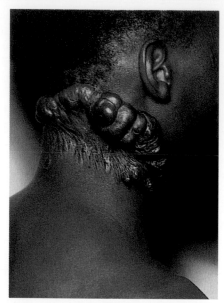

Fig. 1.9 Keloid scarring. (Reproduced with kind permission from Dr C. Lawrence, Wound Healing Research Unit, Cardiff.)

Abnormal Scarring

Hypertrophic and keloid scarring are types of abnormal scarring caused by excessive collagen formation. In these scars the collagen fibre organization differs from that seen in normal scar tissue. Hypertrophic scars have nodular structures, whereas keloids do not.[46]

Hypertrophic Scars

Hypertrophic scars (Fig. 1.8) are more common in the young, following traumatic injuries and large burns. In surgical wounds they tend to follow the line of the incision and occur shortly after injury. Prolonged or disrupted cytokine activity following the inflammatory phase of healing has been proposed[14] as the stimulus for hypertrophic scar formation. The nodular structure of hypertrophic scars can be likened to that of an onion skin, where the collagen is arranged in parallel sheets.[46] The collagen within the centre of the nodule is characterized by the presence of fine, disorganized fibrils, much like the collagen organization in early granulation tissue. Careful placement of incisions along Langer's lines[47] and fine, absorbable suture material can often avoid excessive scar formation.

Keloid Scars

Keloid scars often occur some time after healing. They are characterized by scar tissue around the site of the wound (Fig. 1.9). This is due to an increase in collagen synthesis and lysis and is also thought to be linked to the melanocyte-stimulating hormone[48]; it is very common in people with pigmented skin. Keloids lack the nodular structure of hypertrophic scars. Here, collagen fibres are arranged in thick bands comprising numerous fine collagen fibrils that run parallel to each other.[46] Often these scars are larger than the wound itself. Following excision of the keloid, it is likely to recur.

Atrophic Scars

Atrophic scars are weak and thin and resemble stretch marks. Although there is little to explain why they occur (as with the other abnormalities), they are more common in certain individuals than others.

Contractures

Contractures occur when there is excessive wound contraction and are most common in skin not tethered to underlying deep fascia or other structures. They often occur over joints, impairing their mobility.[4] Fibroblasts constrict the neighbouring collagen fibres surrounding them,[15] causing contracture of the tissue. Again, it is not fully understood why this occurs in some people and not others but it is important when planning surgical procedures to consider the effect of contraction, especially in areas around the joints.

Local Wound Assessment

Accurate assessment of a wound depends on the nurse's ability to recognize normal and abnormal healing. In addition, understanding the aetiology and any underlying pathology will guide the nurse towards planning appropriate care. Local wound assessment includes sutured wounds healing by primary intention and granulating wounds healing by secondary intention.

SUTURED WOUNDS

In many surgical procedures the surgeon can bring the edges of the wound together by using sutures, staples and glues to affect primary closure.[47] Suitable procedures are:

- clean surgical procedures
- procedures that result in little loss of tissue
- procedures where tissues can be brought together without causing tension.

The length of time a sutured wound will take to heal depends not only on the general health of the individual but also on the site of the incision. Where the sutured area has a good blood supply (e.g., wounds on the head and neck), healing may be completed within 3 days. Other sites may take up to 14 days. Sutures should be removed as soon as possible following healing to minimize scarring but must be left in for long enough to prevent the wound dehiscing.

Dressings

A great deal of debate has ensued about whether sutured wounds need to be dressed. It is usual for a simple dressing to be applied in theatre (e.g., an absorbent island dressing) and then removed 24–48 hours later, but this practice varies significantly and people should follow local guidelines.

Postoperative Observations

The wound dressing and the surrounding area should be observed at least once every 24 hours and whenever the patient complains of pain or discomfort. Newer

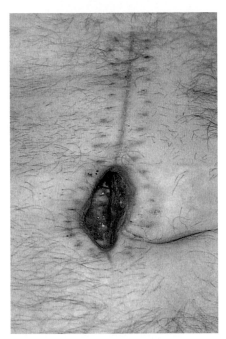

Fig. 1.10 Partial wound breakdown following cholecystectomy.

transparent dressings allow visualization of the wound without the need to remove the dressing.

In a normal, healthy, sutured wound, some degree of inflammation, swelling and redness is to be expected around 2–3 days postoperatively. This demonstrates that the wound is in the inflammatory phase of healing. However, observation should be maintained for the clinical signs of infection, which are:

- generalized malaise and the patient complaining of feeling unwell
- pyrexia and tachycardia
- wound beginning to discharge
- the area surrounding the wound becoming red, sore, swollen and indurated
- on removal of a suture, pus is discharged
- partial wound breakdown following removal of sutures (Fig. 1.10).

GRANULATING WOUNDS

Exudate Production

The amount of exudate an open wound produces can vary tremendously throughout the healing phase (Fig. 1.11). In the immediate postoperative period, surgically created cavities can produce large amounts of

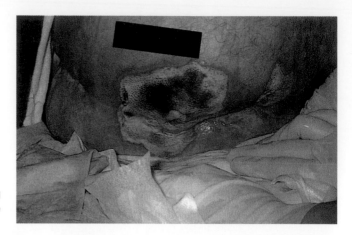

Fig. 1.11 Excessive exudate being produced by a large sacral pressure ulcer. Note the maceration of the skin surrounding the wound.

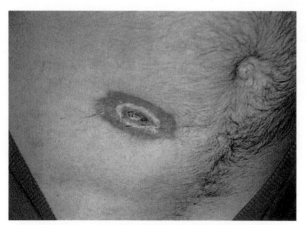

Fig. 1.12 A dry wound bed on an abdominal wall wound.

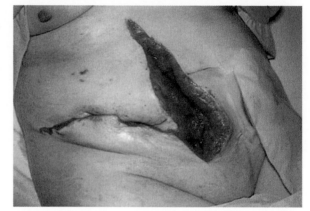

Fig. 1.13 Pregranulation. An abdominal wound 3 days after surgery.

wound exudate. It is usual for exudate production to diminish throughout the healing phase as a wound becomes smaller. However, wounds will continue to ooze small amounts of exudate until complete re-epithelialization has occurred.

On the other hand, wound beds that are dry are not considered to be healthy and will need careful assessment and documentation in preparation for intervention (Fig. 1.12).

Appearance of the Wound Bed

The appearance of the wound bed indicates both the stage of healing and the health of the wound.

A newly created surgical cavity often appears red and raw and has adipose tissue or muscle at the base of the wound. This appearance is normal during the first

2 weeks of healing, prior to granulation tissue being formed (Fig. 1.13).

Healthy granulation tissue appears at around 14 days and persists throughout the healing phase. It is pale pink or yellow and has a bumpy or 'cobblestone' appearance. Healthy granulation tissue is firm to touch, painless and does not bleed.

Towards the end of healing, new epithelium covers the surface of the wound. It is pale pink in colour and is usually seen at the edges of the wound, gradually creeping toward the middle to cover the wound completely (Fig. 1.14).

Slough

Slough is most commonly seen lining the base of chronic wounds such as leg ulcers and pressure ulcers

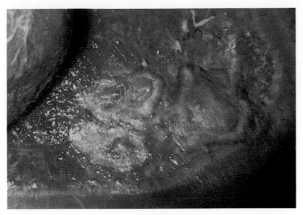

Fig. 1.14 Epithelialization.

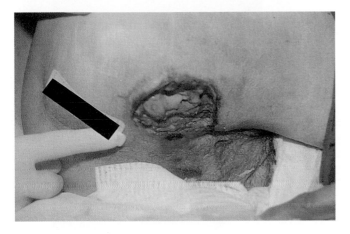

Fig. 1.15 Sloughy tissue on the wound bed of a grade IV pressure ulcer with underlying extensive tissue damage.

(Fig. 1.15). It is yellow, white or grey in appearance and consists of dead, devitalized tissue, fibrin, bacteria, leucocytes, cell debris, serous exudate and DNA.[49] Slough may cover the wound bed totally or partially, with patches of healthy tissue. It can be dry or moist and is characterized by being firmly adherent to the base of the wound. While removal of slough is often recommended, there is a lack of evidence that its removal improves the rate of healing in venous leg ulcers.[50]

Necrotic Tissue

Necrotic tissue is often seen in conjunction with slough. Necrotic tissue is black or blackish-green in appearance, but unlike slough it is completely dead tissue (Fig. 1.16). Necrotic tissue can be hard and leathery in appearance or soft and moist. As with slough, it is firmly stuck to the wound bed and consists of desiccated, compressed layers of tissue. Typically, dead subcutaneous tissue is associated with softer necrosis, and muscle and skin death with thicker, more leathery necrosis, and is often seen in burn injuries.[49] According to the European Wound Management Association, debridement is the act of removing necrotic material, eschar, devitalized tissue, serocrusts, infected tissue, hyperkeratosis, slough, pus, haematomas, foreign bodies, debris, bone fragments or any other type of bioburden from a wound with the objective to promote wound healing.[49]

Hypergranulation

Occasionally re-epithelialization fails to take place owing to the presence of excessive granulation tissue (hypergranulation or proud flesh). Epithelial migration

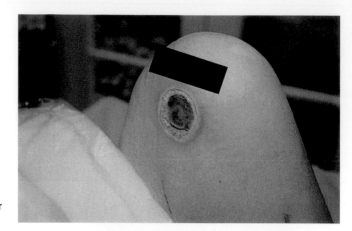

Fig. 1.16 Necrotic tissue covering a pressure ulcer on the inner aspect of the knee.

cannot continue over hypergranulation and this tissue needs to be flattened to effect complete healing through re-epithelialization.

WOUND SHAPE

It is important to recognize the importance of wound shape and its effect on healing. Ideally, surgically created cavities should be boat shaped or saucer shaped, with evenly sloping sides. This allows free drainage of wound secretions and enables easy dressing of the wound. Many chronic wounds, especially pressure ulcers, are irregularly shaped with undermining pockets, tracts and sinuses. Where these are present, drainage of wound secretions is inadequate, encouraging wound infection. Poor wound shape also restricts the range of dressing materials that can be used. Occasionally wound shape is so poor and progress towards healing is so slow that surgical revision may be needed to give the wound more regular contours.

WOUND SIZE

Wound size can be difficult to measure accurately and there are several methods of achieving this, including a simple ruler technique, acetate tracing, sophisticated three-dimensional imaging and digital planimetry. Whatever technique is used, it is important to be consistent as different methods will give slightly different results. Ruler technique, while providing some indication of wound size, overestimates size; acetate tracing is more reliable and accurate and is comparable to planimetry, particularly for wounds <10 cm². This method is inexpensive, easy to use and provides a visual representation to the patient and the clinician.[51]

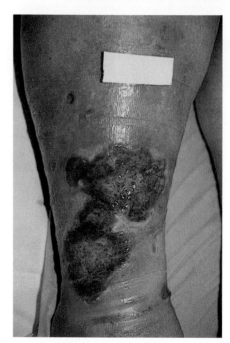

Fig. 1.17 An infected venous leg ulcer showing unhealthy granulation tissue and maceration of the surrounding skin.

WOUND INFECTION

Wound infection can occur at any time during the healing phase and in all types of wounds (Figs 1.17 and 1.18). All wounds are colonized with bacteria that do not necessarily delay or affect healing; however, pathogenic organisms growing in large numbers are likely to produce wound infection.[29] Some patients are more vulnerable to infection than others and it is the relationship between the susceptibility

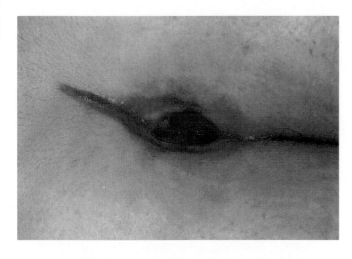

Fig. 1.18 Infection occurring during healing of a pilonidal sinus wound. Note the unhealthy appearance of the granulation tissue. An anaerobic organism has been cultured from this wound.

of the host and the virulence of the pathogen that dictates the severity of the infection.[52]

Pathogenic organisms that commonly cause wound infection are listed below.

Aerobic Bacteria

Aerobic bacteria thrive in the presence of oxygen but do not necessarily depend upon it.

- *Staphylococcus aureus* is carried by around 30% of the population and causes many hospital-acquired wound infections.
- *Staphylococcus epidermidis* is found in large quantities on the intact skin of individuals. It is present in the air and in dust, being constantly shed by the skin and counts are especially high when people are frequently moving around in enclosed spaces.
- Methicillin-resistant *Staphylococcus aureus* (MRSA) has been a cause of hospital-acquired infection for many years. With the discovery of penicillin, serious outbreaks of hospital-acquired infections were brought under control. Unfortunately, *S. aureus* quickly developed resistance to penicillin. The emergence of MRSA was reported in 1961[53] and it has been causing problems ever since, especially in intensive care units and elderly care wards.[54] Methods of spread include the unwashed hands of doctors and nurses, contact with heavily contaminated families and surfaces, and airborne spread from infected patients.[54,55]

A high incidence of sepsis and serious complications occurs in seriously ill patients, including those who have suffered burns or who are immunocompromised.

- Beta-haemolytic streptococci are found in around 5% of the population and more commonly in those suffering from acute tonsillitis. In burns and plastic surgery units these bacteria cause infection under skin grafts and can lead to the death of the graft.
- *Escherichia coli* and *Proteus* are normal bowel flora. These bacteria can be spread by hand contamination or by local approximation of the perineum to the wound. Sacral pressure ulcers are prime candidates for such contamination, especially if the patient is incontinent of faeces. Occasionally spillage may occur during intestinal surgery that contaminates the surgical incision.
- *Klebsiella* and *Pseudomonas* (Fig. 1.19) are found in moist conditions although they are also normal bowel commensals. Because they are free living these bacteria can easily contaminate lotions and antiseptics.

Anaerobic Bacteria

Anaerobic bacteria thrive in the absence of oxygen and so are suited to the conditions found in the bowel and in soil.

- *Bacteroides* are present in large numbers in the bowels of healthy individuals. In pilonidal sinus excisions these micro-organisms are responsible

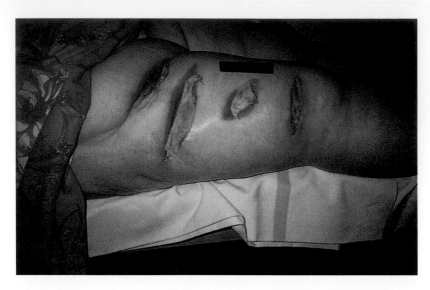

Fig. 1.19 Abscess excision sites infected with *Pseudomonas*. Note the blue-green discharge characteristic of *Pseudomonas*.

for an infection rate of around 20%, owing to the close proximity of these wounds to the anus. Leakage during bowel surgery can cause peritonitis.

- *Clostridium perfringens* is a potentially fatal organism. This spore-bearing organism is present in the bowel and in soil and when it contaminates a wound it can cause gas gangrene. Poorly perfused wound sites such as amputation stumps or deep contaminated traumatic cavities are especially at risk.
- *Clostridium tetani* is another spore-bearing organism that infects wounds that have been exposed to dirt or soil where these bacteria are commonly found, causing tetanus in the unprotected individual.

Susceptible Patients

Patients who are susceptible to developing wound infection include:

- immunocompromised or patients with a debilitating illness
- patients with devitalized tissue in their wound
- patients with a haematoma in their wound
- patients with a poor blood supply to the wound
- patients who are at risk of contamination of their wound, e.g., through dementia or incontinence
- older patients
- obese patients

- patients who are shaved preoperatively or who stay in hospital for longer than 7 days preoperatively.[12,29,56]

Possible routes of infection in patients with wounds are shown in Fig. 1.20.

Possible Causes of Wound Infection

Wound infection does not occur in all situations where pathogenic organisms are found but depends on the number of pathogens, their virulence and the host's resistance to infection.[57] It occurs when the physiological balance is upset, either because the host's defences are lowered or because the microorganism is particularly virulent.[52] This situation causes failure by the host to control micro-organism growth, evidenced by localized infection which, if unchecked, can lead to deep-seated and more severe infection.[52]

Clinical Signs of Infection

Infected granulation tissue (Fig. 1.21) has an appearance characterized by:

- flimsy, friable granulation tissue
- superficial bridging within the wound
- spontaneous bleeding or bleeding on light contact
- pain or discomfort within the wound
- delayed healing or wound enlargement
- offensive wound exudate
- pus formation

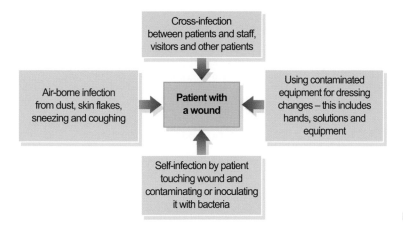

Fig. 1.20 Sources of infection in hospital.

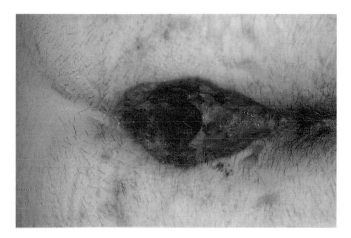

Fig. 1.21 A pilonidal sinus wound illustrating the clinical signs of infection. (Reproduced with kind permission from the *Journal of Wound Care*, London.)

- cellulitis or inflammation in the tissues surrounding the wound.[12]

Infection in primary wound closure is characterized by:

- redness, inflammation and induration of the tissues surrounding the wound (not associated with the immediate postoperative inflammatory phase of healing, which is a normal phenomenon occurring around days 1–3 following surgery)
- partial wound breakdown accompanied by a discharge of pus or haemoserous fluid
- pain, throbbing and heat in the wound area and surrounding tissues.

It is usually necessary to take a sample of wound exudate or discharge for culture and sensitivity by the bacteriology laboratory. Identifying the organism causing the wound infection, together with its sensitivity to an antibiotic, facilitates early treatment of the wound infection. Nurses should consider what information they require from the laboratory and make this implicit on the laboratory forms. In addition, attention needs to be paid to swabbing technique, which should include using an aseptic technique and gathering as much exudate as possible without contaminating the sterile swab with skin flora. The swab should be sent to the laboratory as soon as possible, within 24 hours at the latest, using a transport medium where appropriate.

Assessment of the Environment

The final step in this organized approach considers the physical and social environment in which the individual is being cared for. The recent document from the European Wound Management Association, *Home Care–Wound Care*, provides some recommendations for caring for the individual in their own home and the challenges therein.[58]

Summary

This chapter has covered aspects that need to be considered when assessing any patient with a wound, whether simple or complex. Before proceeding to the next chapter, reflect on these aspects:

- Assessment of the individual
  - Recognizing the stages of normal healing
  - Recognizing abnormal healing processes
  - Wound healing by primary or secondary intention
- Factors that affect healing
  - Intrinsic
  - Extrinsic
- Assessment of the wound
  - Sutured or granulating
  - Shape and size
  - Infection
- Assessment of the environment
  - Hospital based
  - Community based
  - Caregivers

The way in which all these aspects can be used in an organized framework is discussed in the next chapter.

FURTHER READING

Bale S, Harding K, Leaper D. *An Introduction to Wounds*. London: Emap Healthcare Ltd; 2000.

Bryant RA. *Acute and Chronic Wounds: Nursing Management*. 4th ed. St Louis, Missouri: Mosby; 2012.

Falanga V. *Cutaneous Wound Healing*. London: Martin Dunitz; 2001.

Leaper D, Harding K. *Wounds: Biology and Management*. Oxford: Oxford Medical Publications; 1998.

REFERENCES

1. Gethin G, Killeen F, Devane D. Heterogeneity of wound outcome measures in RCTs of treatments for VLUs: a systematic review. *J Wound Care*. 2015;24(5):211–212.
2. Lazaro-Martinez JL, Conde-Montero E, Alvarez-Vazquez JC, et al. Preliminary experience of an expert panel using triangle wound assessment for the evaluation of chronic wounds. *J Wound Care*. 2018;27(11):790–796.
3. Schultz G, Sibbald G, Falanga V, et al. Wound bed preparation: a systematic approach to wound management. *Wound Repair Regen*. 2003;11:1–28.
4. Locono J, Ehrlich HP, Gottrup F, Leaper D. The biology of wound healing. In: Leaper D, Harding K, eds. *Wounds: Biology and Management*. Oxford: Oxford Medical Publications; 1998.
5. Gethin G. Understanding the inflammatory process in wound healing. *Br J Community Nurs*. 2012;(suppl):S17–S18.
6. Greener B, Hughes A, Bannister N, Douglass J. Proteases and pH in chronic wounds. *J Wound Care*. 2005;14(2):59–61.
7. Slavin J. Wound healing: pathophysiology *Surgery*. 1999;17(4):1–5.
8. Lingen M, Nickoloff B. Role of immunocytes, cytokines and angiogenesis in wound healing. In: Falanga V, ed. *Cutaneous Wound Healing*. London: Martin Dunitz; 2001.
9. Hart J. Inflammation 1: its role in the healing of acute wounds. *J Wound Care*. 2002;11(6):205–209.
10. Hart J. Inflammation 2: its role in the healing of chronic wounds. *J Wound Care*. 2002;11(7):245–249.
11. Wysocki A. Anatomy and physiology of skin and soft tissue. In: Bryant R, Nix D, eds. *Acute and Chronic Wounds: Nursing management*. 4th ed. St. Louis, Missouri: Mosby; 2012.
12. Cutting K, White R. Criteria for identifying wound infection-revisited. *Ostomy Wound Manag*. 2005;51:28–34.
13. Neal MS. Angiogenesis: is it the key to controlling the healing process? *J Wound Care*. 2001;10(7):281–287.
14. O'Kane S. Wound remodelling and scarring. *J Wound Care*. 2002;11(8):296–299.
15. Cho M, Hunt TK. The overall approach to wounds. In: Falanga V, ed. *Cutaneous Wound Healing*. London: Martin Dunitz; 2001.
16. Shanmugam VK, Fernandez SJ, Evans KK, et al. Postoperative wound dehiscence: predictors and associations. *Wound Repair Regen*. 2015;23(2):184–190.
17. Smith CT, Katz MG, Foley D, et al. Incidence and risk factors of incisional hernia formation following abdominal organ transplantation. *Surg Endosc*. 2015;29(2):398–404.
18. Franks P, Barker J, Collier M, et al. Management of patients with venous leg ulcers: challenges and current best practice. *J Wound Care*. 2016;25:S1.
19. Hunter JA. Clinical Dermatology. Oxford: Blackwell Science; 1995.
20. Sgonc R, Gruber J. Age-related aspects of cutaneous wound healing: a mini-review. *Gerontol*. 2013;59(2):159–164.
21. Jockenhöfer F, Gollnick H, Herberger K, et al. Aetiology, comorbidities and cofactors of chronic leg ulcers: retrospective evaluation of 1000 patients from 10 specialised dermatological wound care centers in Germany. *Int Wound J*. 2016;13(5):821–828.
22. Guo S, DiPietro LA. Factors affecting wound healing. *J Dental Res*. 2010;89(3):219–229.
23. Egydio F, Tomimori J, Tufik S, Andersen ML. Does sleep deprivation and morphine influence wound healing? *Med Hypotheses*. 2011;77(3):353–355.
24. Padgett DA, Marucha PT, Sheridan JF. Restraint stress slows cutaneous wound healing in mice. *Brain Behav Immun*. 1998;12(1):64–73.
25. McGloin H, Devane D, McIntosh C, Winkley K, Gethin G. Psychological interventions for treating and preventing recurrence of foot ulcers in people with diabetes. *Cochrane Database of Syst Rev*. 2017;(10):CD012835.
26. Dealey C. The management of patients with wounds. In: Dealey C, ed. *The Care of Wounds*. Oxford: Blackwell; 1999.
27. Rodgers S. The patient facing surgery. In: Alexander M, Fawcett J, Runciman P, eds. *Nursing Practice: Hospital and Home, the Adult*. Edinburgh: Churchill Livingstone; 1999.
28. Probst S, Arber A, Faithfull S. Malignant fungating wounds: the meaning of living in an unbounded body. *Eur J Oncol Nurs*. 2013;17(1):38–45.
29. Leaper D, Harding K. The problems of wound infection. In: Bale S, Harding K, Leaper D, eds. *An Introduction to Wounds*. London: Emap Healthcare Ltd.; 2000.
30. Kopelman P, Lennard-Jones J. Nutrition and patients: a doctor's responsibility. *Clin Med*. 2002;2(5):391–394.
31. McLaren SM. Nutrition and wound healing. *J Wound Care*. 1992;1(3):45–55.
32. Stotts N. Nutritional assessment and support. In: Bryant R, Nix

D, eds. *Acute and Chronic Wounds, Current Management Options.* 4th ed. St. Louis, Missouri: Elsevier; 2012.

33. Dickerson J. The problem of hospital-induced malnutrition. *Nurs Times.* 1995;91(4):44–45.
34. McWhirter JP, Pennington CR. Incidence and recognition of malnutrition in hospital. *BMJ.* 1994;308(6934):945–948.
35. Gray D, Cooper P. Nutrition and wound healing: what is the link? *J Wound Care.* 2001;10(3):86–89.
36. EPUAP. Guide to pressure ulcer grading. *EPUAP review.* 2009;3. Available at: http://www.epuap.org/.
37. Pinchcofsky-Devin G. *Nutrition and Wound Healing. 3rd European Conference on advances in wound management.* Harrogate, UK: EMAP Healthcare; 1993.
38. EPUAP. Prevention and treatment of pressure ulcers. 2009 05 02 2019. Available at: http://www.epuap.org.
39. Harris CL, Fraser C. Malnutrition in the institutionalized elderly: the effects on wound healing [corrected]. [published errata appear in Ostomy Wound Manag. 2004;50(11):10] *Ostomy Wound Manag.* 2004;50(10):54–63.
40. Williams L. Assessing patients' nutritional needs in the wound-healing process. *J Wound Care.* 2002;11(6):225–228.
41. Siana JE, Rex S, Gottrup F. The effect of cigarette smoking on wound healing. *Scand J Plast Reconstr Surg Hand Surg.* 1989;23(3):207–209.
42. Waldrop J, Doughty D. Wound-healing physiology. In: Bryant R, Nix D, eds. *Acute and Chronic Wounds: Current Management Concepts.* 4th ed. St. Louis, Missouri: Elsevier; 2012.
43. Sorensen LT. Wound healing and infection in surgery. The clinical impact of smoking and smoking cessation. A systematic review and meta-analysis. *Wound Repair Regen.* 2012;20(5). A113–A.
44. Fu XL, Ding H, Miao WW, Chen HL. Association between cigarette smoking and diabetic foot healing: a systematic review and meta analysis. *Int J Low Extrem Wounds.* 2018;17(4):247–257.
45. Grocott P, Gethin G, Probst S. Skin problems in palliative care – nursing aspects. In: Cherny N, Fallon M, Kaasa S, Portenoy R, Currow D, eds. *Oxford Textbook of Palliative Medicine.* Oxford University Press; 2015.
46. Ehrlich HP, Gottrup F. Experimental models in wound healing.

In: Leaper D, Harding K, eds. *Wounds: Biology and Management.* Oxford: Oxford Medical Publications; 1998.
47. Leaper D, Gottrup F. Surgical wounds. In: Leaper D, Harding K, eds. *Wounds: Biology and Management.* Oxford: Oxford Medical Publications; 1998.
48. Eisenbeiss W, Peter FW, Bakhtiari C, Frenz C. Hypertrophic scars and keloids. *J Wound Care.* 1998;7(5):255–257.
49. Strohal R. The EWMA document: debridement. *J Wound Care.* 2013;22(1):5.
50. Gethin G, Cowman S, Kolbach DN. Debridement for venous leg ulcers. *Cochrane Database of Systematic Reviews.* 2015(9):CD008599.
51. Gethin G, Cowman S. Wound measurement comparing the use of acetate tracings and Visitrak digital planimetry. *J Clin Nurs.* 2006;15(4):422–427.
52. Leaper DJ, Schultz G, Carville K, Fletcher J, Swanson T, Drake R. Extending the TIME concept: what have we learned in the past 10 years? *Int Wound J.* 2012;9:1–19.
53. Jevans M. "Celbenin"-resistant staphylococci. *Br Med J.* 1961;1:124.
54. Poovelikunnel TT, Gethin G, Solanki D, McFadden E, Codd M, Humphreys H. Randomized controlled trial of honey versus mupirocin to decolonize patients with nasal colonization of meticillin-resistant *Staphylococcus aureus. J Hosp Infect.* 2018;98(2):141–148.
55. Poovelikunnel T, Gethin G, Humphreys H. Mupirocin resistance: clinical implications and potential alternatives for the eradication of MRSA. *J Antimicrob Chemother.* 2015;70(10):2681–2692.
56. Lipsky BA, Dryden M, Gottrup F, Nathwani D, Seaton RA, Stryja J. Antimicrobial stewardship in wound care: a position paper from the British Society for Antimicrobial Chemotherapy and European Wound Management Association. *J Antimicrob Chemother.* 2016;71(11):3026–3035.
57. Gardner S, Frantz R, Doebbeling B. The validity of the clinical signs and symptoms used to identify localized chronic wound infection. *Wound Repair Regen.* 2001;9(3):178–186.
58. Probst S, Seppanen S, Gethin G, Gerber V, Hopkins A, Rimdeika R. EWMA document home care–wound care. *J Wound Care.* 2014;23(5):S1–S44.

MCQS

1 *The recommended daily intake of protein is:*
a. 10–15 g per kg daily
b. 10–15 g daily
c. 1–1.5 g per kg daily
d. 15–20 g per day

2 *Fibrin clot is formed in which stage of wound healing?*
a. Inflammatory stage
b. Haemostasis stage
c. Proliferative stage
d. Maturation stage

3 *Which type of collagen is laid down in the maturation stage?*
a. Type 3 collagen
b. Type 8 collagen
c. Type 3 and 8 collagen
d. None of the above

Chapter 2

Assessing and Planning Individualized Care

Sinéad Hahessy

Highlights

- This chapter gives an overview of nursing theory and the basis of nursing models which are used as a framework for assessing patients with wounds
- This chapter addresses the theory–practice gap
- This chapter discusses Peplau's model, Orem's self-care model, Roy's adaptation model, Riehl interaction model and Roper, Logan and Tierney's model

Key Issues

Nursing models are classified and outlined as follows:
- Developmental
  - Peplau's model
  - Orem's model
- Systems
  - Roy's model
  - Roper, Logan and Tierney's model
- Interaction
  - Riehl's model
  Goal setting and outcomes are also covered.

Introduction

Assessing a patient with a wound can prove to be difficult, especially for the inexperienced practitioner. However, careful selection of a theory and model of nursing to guide assessment, and ultimately the care trajectory of the patient, is primarily underpinned by personal and socio-political, spiritual and educational influences on the nurse.

There are many ways in which nurses practically assess their patients: some use a medical model framework and others use a nursing model. In order to use a nursing model, nurses must understand the basis of the model. In the right circumstances nursing models can provide a clear framework for practitioners to follow, as well as providing an optimum level of care for the patient.

This chapter explains some of the theory that underpins popular and universally recognized nursing models and discusses the type of patient they might be best suited for.

When using an organized framework to identify patient problems, it is important that clear goals and outcomes are identified. The setting of goals and outcomes is explained using examples of particular wound types.

Using a Nursing Model to Assess Individuals

Before using a nursing model, it is important that the nurse understands the nursing theory that underpins it. Often this vital step is overlooked or superficially understood, as models are frequently introduced via the curriculum of a college of nursing or on a regional basis; for example, throughout the clinical areas within an NHS trust.

THEORETICAL BASIS OF MODELS

Since the introduction of nursing models in the 1950s, healthcare systems have undergone numerous changes along with professional developments in clinical nursing practice and the expansion of the role of the nurse. However, one of the major complaints still heard from practitioners is that often nursing theory has little or no relevance to clinical practice. Because models are often imposed or embedded in the culture of a clinical unit, nurses do not have the flexibility to discover how a model fits into their line of practice or which model might be most effective. It is imperative that wound care nurses aim to develop a professional aptitude and competence in discerning which model to utilize for patients with different types of wounds.

The practice of nursing has evolved in response to external and internal drivers such as government policy, advances in the professional accreditation of nurses and globalization, including economic upheaval. The relentless nature of change has required nursing to readdress its philosophical basis, most pertinently in the fundamental areas of care, dignity and ensuring individualized care. In 2013, the Francis Report[1] highlighted the crisis related to erosion of the core values in nursing philosophy. The very essence of nursing has recently been a central focus in various media reports, where the question of 'What has happened to compassion?'[2] blatantly interrogates the fundamental nature of nursing. The emphasis on care requires that nurses re-examine their core values.

Nursing models and theories function to provide a rationale and structure for nursing care.[3] However, in busy and demanding environments these concepts are often disregarded.[4] This amplifies the theory–practice gap. Haugh[5] has argued that the theory–practice gap should be observed as a positive reflection on the dynamic nature of nursing and that theory progresses in a quicker fashion than clinical practice. Remedies to overcome the theory–practice gap require an emphasis on more appropriate education with regard to philosophy, research and practice development and the relationship between theoretical approaches to care. McKenna[15] challenges practitioners to interpret and analyse established theories about their practice where theories have not or cannot be subject to empirical testing.

Wound management is a practical subject that can be used as a focus for the use of a model while drawing continually on the biological and behavioural scientific knowledge that underpins its practice (Fig. 2.1). Chronic wounds are usually indicative of underlying systemic disease and are often viewed, in clinical terms, as being lower in priority to the main disease. Wound care is often conducted in interdisciplinary contexts and many services may be involved in the patient's

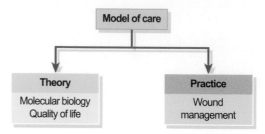

Fig. 2.1 Wound management theory. (Adapted from Akinsanya JA. The uses of theories in nursing. *Nursing Times*. 1984;80(14):59–60, with permission.)

TABLE 2.1 Common Physical and Psychological Issues in Patients with Wounds	
Physical Issues	**Psychological Issues**
Pain	Fear
Odour	Shame
Infection	Inconvenience
Exudate	Isolation
Bleeding/itching	Lack of independence
Discomfort	Altered body image
	Low self-esteem
	Loss of function

treatment, often resulting in communication failure at different points of the journey. Lack of continuity of care and lack of planning for wound care, along with inconsistent patient education and information, often leaves patients confused about many aspects of their care. The European Wound Management Association (EWMA) has identified a range of physical and psychological issues that patients with wounds usually encounter, as outlined in Table 2.1,[6] demonstrating how complex wound care issues can become.

The consensus documents *Optimising wellbeing in people living with a wound*[7] and *Managing wounds as a team*[8] have discussed the evolution of domains of practice aligned to wound care, which are underpinned by the need for a paradigm shift. The domains focus on prevention of death, improving quality of life, recovery, ensuring a positive experience for the patient and maintaining a safe environment. The paradigm shift in wound care encompasses an approach to wound care that (a) emphasizes collaborative practice, (b) is primarily holistic, (c) is focused on the macro context of health and (d) the patient is central in deciding the care trajectory. Wound care is a complex field of practice and the plan of care usually extends across assessment, diagnosis, therapeutics, prevention and prognosis.

Using a nursing model as a framework can help practitioners bring structure to what may appear to be a bewildering array of problems, theories, abstract concepts and haphazard treatments. Models are constructed on the assumption that patient-centred care is in use and even where the 'named nurse' system is apparently functioning, staff shortages, stress and heavy workloads will result in a degree of task allocation, which abandons the notion of using philosophy and theory. In certain circumstances, a nursing model may need to be set aside in favour of a system that prioritizes patients' needs, which are assessed and planned on a less formal basis. This informal method of care is often conducted by 'experienced' nurses who feel they do not need a designated model but set their own framework through which they deliver care to the patient. This informal, trial and error, unsystematic way of working is very difficult to pass on to others as it is often based on intuitive and ritualistic care that has little theoretical foundation.

Theories and models of nursing address four concepts:

- the individual
- society or the environment of care
- health
- nursing, its nature and role.

Deductive or Inductive Approach

Models are based on either a deductive or an inductive approach. These terms are derived from the physical sciences, as is the concept of using models, which originally were physical representations of physical objects. Later on, the behavioural sciences adopted the use of models to predict behaviour.

The laws of physical science were established through the formulation of hypotheses which were then formally tested by experimental methods. This is known as the deductive method; it relies heavily on controlling the variables under study and is not always suitable for the behavioural sciences such as psychology and sociology. During the 1960s sociologists found that the generation of theory was better achieved by observation of practice and behaviour. This is the inductive approach to theory generation which has been found to be very suitable for nursing research. It

TABLE 2.2	A Patient's Problems
Activities of Living have been Grouped According to their Degree of Correspondence to Physiological Systems	
Activity of Living	**Problem Statements**
Maintaining a safe environment	Risk of self-injury (P)
Communicating	Diminished verbal response Anxiety, depression Accent
Breathing	Cough Infected sputum Pain Dyspnoea Cigarette smoking
Eating and drinking	Anorexia Dehydration Poor dentition Oral infection (P)
Elimination	Renal failure (P) Renal infection (P) Constipation (P)
Personal cleansing and dressing	Inability or unwillingness to care for self Excessive perspiration
Controlling body temperature	Dehydration (P)
Mobilizing	Immobility Pressure sores (P) Deep vein thrombosis Exacerbation of chest infection
Working and playing Expressing sexuality Sleeping	
Dying	Non-acceptance of nature of disease (P)

P, Potential problem.
(Reproduced with permission from Roper N, Logan WW, Tierney AJ. *Using a Model for Nursing*. Edinburgh: Churchill Livingstone; 1983.)

also facilitated the move away from the medical model of care, as medical knowledge is largely based on the deductive method of theory generation. This shift has not been an easy or comfortable move for many nurses and often nursing models are still used as medical models. This is highlighted in Table 2.2, which is an example of Roper's activities of living model[9] in use on a medical ward. The problems identified are largely medical conditions and symptoms, such as renal failure and dehydration.

CLASSIFICATION OF MODELS

Models can be classified according to their underpinning theory as follows:

- developmental
- systems
- interaction.

However, many models will not be totally illuminated by one underlying philosophy but will contain aspects of two or even all three theories. This can often lead to confusion when trying to establish the theoretical underpinnings of a particular model. The models used in this book are categorized according to their *primary* focus.

Developmental Models

Developmental models focus on theories of development or change. These theories centre on how a person is developing and how nursing can help when normal development is threatened or impaired.

In the developmental process, stages follow a predictable course and proceed in an orderly fashion, even towards illness or death. Development covers not just the physical but psychological and social processes as well. Developmental models focus on helping the patient attain new developmental goals or re-establishing a developmental stage from which the patient has regressed. The two best-known models in this category are those of Peplau[10] and Orem.[11]

Peplau's Model

Hildegard Peplau was one of the first American theorists to address the changing needs of nursing.[10] She recognized that often the care that a patient *needs* may well be different from what the patient *wants*.

Believing that nursing was based on the formation of a relationship between nurse and patient, she stressed the importance of the roles and phases through which nurse and patient pass during the interpersonal process. The first purpose of the nurse is to ensure survival of the patient, the second is to help them understand and come to terms with their health problems. For example, when a patient with diabetes mellitus has a foot amputated because of ischaemia, the first concern of the nurse is control of the diabetes and infection. Both conditions, unchecked, can potentially be life threatening. The nurse's second concern is to help the patient come to terms with the loss of a foot and learn how to mobilize again.

In moving towards health, the patient experiences four phases: orientation, identification, exploration and resolution. These four phases correspond to the four phases of the nursing process:

- *Orientation* (assessment): nurse learns the nature of the difficulty the patient is experiencing; development of mutual trust; problem identification.
- *Identification* (planning): recognition by the patient of the formulation of the nurse–patient relationship; nurse plans appropriate intervention.
- *Exploitation* (implementation): patient recognizes and responds to services offered by the nurse; interpersonal relationship is fully established; both nurse and patient move towards mutual goals.
- *Resolution* (evaluation): health problem resolved or improved; nursing input no longer required or at minimal level; patient returns to independence; new goals or existing developmental stage re-established.

Peplau's model has no particular framework or form of record keeping to be used during the assessment phase. She advocates the use of the acronym 'SOAP':

S – the *subjective experience* as described by the patient

O – *objective observation* made by the nurse

A – *formal assessment* and identification of problems (based on S and O)

P – *plan* of action.

For an example, see Case study 4.3.

Orem's Self-Care Model

Dorothea Orem's framework has been classified previously as a systems model[12] and latterly as a self-care model. However, Fawcett[13] agreed that Orem's model demonstrates strong characteristics of a developmental model. The model emphasizes the concept of self-care, where people take responsibility for their own healthcare, which is provided, where possible, by friends and family. The model rejects the passive role of the patient and is more in tune with contemporary nursing, which allows patients to participate in their own care.

The characteristics of growth, development and maturation are classified in Orem's model as self-care requisites and can be described as basic human needs. They are:

- sufficient intake of air
- sufficient intake of water
- sufficient intake of food
- satisfactory eliminatory functions
- activity balanced with rest
- time spent alone balanced with time spent with others
- prevention of danger to self
- being normal.

Two further self-care requisites are described.

- *Developmental self-care requisites:* these may affect the universal self-care requisites according to the stage of development of the individual or the environment in which the individual lives.
- *Health deviation self-care requisites:* ill health or disability may necessitate a change in self-care behaviour.

Self-care is possible when individuals are able to cope with the demands placed upon them. When these demands become too great or the individual's ability to cope decreases, then an imbalance occurs, causing a 'self-care deficit'.

Assessment using Orem's model should be carried out in two stages.

Stage 1 – establishing *if* there is a self-care deficit.

Stage 2 – if there is, establishing *why* there is a self-care deficit. Is it because the patient lacks knowledge, skill or motivation, or has a limited range of behaviour?

Having identified a self-care deficit, the nurse should plan – with the patient where possible – the goals of care. The nurse must decide whether the intervention will be:

- wholly compensatory, i.e., the nurse acts for the patient completely
- partly compensatory, i.e., certain aspects of care are shared by patient and nurse
- educative–developmental, i.e., the nurse gives the patient the necessary knowledge or skills to allow self-care.

The level at which the patient is involved in planning care will depend on the patient's physical and mental

---

Case Study 2.1

Pilonidal Sinus Wound

Steven Jones is a 22-year-old student who has undergone surgery for excision of a pilonidal sinus. He is anxious to return home and to his studies as he has examinations in 6 weeks' time.

The nurse explains verbally how he can change his foam dressing himself. She does not:

enquire if he has any help (partner, parent or friend) who could assist with the dressing change

explain the importance of cleansing his foam 'bung' twice daily

watch Steven doing the dressing change before discharge

explain the importance of personal hygiene and infection control

give any written explanation.

Steven goes home with his dressings; however, without support at home and without any kind of written guidance, he quickly forgets what he has to do. He consequently rings his general practitioner who sends the district nurse to the house to help with the dressing change. The district nurse is annoyed with Steven and the hospital as she feels this to be an unnecessary call, when she has many less able patients to call on. Steven feels stupid and inadequate that he is unable to cope.

---

state but the nurse should always aim to maximize the patient's input where possible. The patient's relatives or carers should be included in this planning as they may be a key factor in helping the patient achieve this potential.

Nursing *intervention* follows the planning stage. Orem has distinguished five methods of implementing the care plan:

1. acting or doing for another
2. guiding another
3. supporting another, physically or psychologically
4. providing an environment that promotes personal development
5. teaching another.

The move from dependence to independence is clear in this model. It must be stressed, however, that giving a patient a task to do without assessing their potential is not self-care and may have dire consequences, as in Case study 2.1. With proper assessment and planning this situation could have been avoided. Can you see why it occurred?

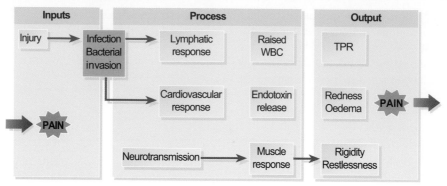

Fig. 2.2 Wound infection – a systems approach. **WBC, white blood cell count; TPR, temperature, pulse, respiration.** (Adapted from Chapman CM. *Theory of Nursing: Practical Application.* London: Harper & Row, 1985, with permission.)

Humanists such as Abraham Maslow[14] and Martha E. Rogers[15] have highlighted the importance of human emotion, known as *affect,* which has a powerful influence on thought processes and human behaviour.[16] Orem's self-care model draws on Maslow's 'hierarchy of needs' theory.[17] The premise is that people are motivated to realise their self-actualization, which can be impeded by physical or psychological decline. The nurse facilitates the patient to realize their potential.

Systems Models

Systems models are characterized by the progression along a lifespan, the examination of the system, its parts and their relationship with each other at a given time.

The major features of systems models are the system and its environment. It is how the system reacts to the environment and maintains its equilibrium that is of major interest. In contrast to developmental models, change is of secondary importance. Systems models are concerned with maintaining a balance along the lifespan; although each part is studied separately, interaction of the parts is most important.

'System' and 'environment' are defined according to the context of study; for example, a system could be a person whose parts are body organs and whose environment is the family.

Systems may be open or closed. An open system is one of continuous inflow and outflow; the outflow becoming the inflow for the next stage of the system and so on. Open systems are therefore influenced by internal and external factors; the less interference from either of these factors, the more smoothly the system will run.

As in the human body, a disturbance in the function of one of the internal subsystems or external factors will produce an imbalance. In order for the body to maintain homeostasis, a new balance has to be achieved. This may be self-regulated, for example the production of insulin for the conversion of glucose to give energy. Outside intervention from medical and nursing staff will be required when the body is unable to regulate an imbalance; for example, when a patient has a wound infection, the initial reaction by the body will be an increase in the number of white blood cells (i.e., a lymphatic response) and also a cardiovascular response, producing the signs and symptoms of infection. With the output the patient experiences pain, which subsequently becomes an input (Fig. 2.2).

Understanding this systems approach will help the nurse to identify priorities of care and provide intervention that will minimize further complications or deterioration. This method of care is proactive rather than reactive, i.e., it deals with a problem before it arises rather than after.

Two models that have a distinct systems approach are Roy's adaptation model[18] and Roper, Logan and Tierney's activities of living model.[9]

Roy's Adaptation Model

Calista Roy began developing this model in the mid-1960s in California. She sees the person as an individual whose behaviour is governed by a set of interrelated biological, psychological and social systems. In order to maintain a balance, individuals are in a constant state of interaction, both within themselves and in their relationship with the outside world. Demands or stressors can be anything experienced in life and how an individual copes or adapts to these will vary from person to person. It is the nurse's ability to identify stressors that will influence the patient's recovery. When the nurse is able to do this, their role should be to promote the patient's ability to adapt and cope with the new demands. However, a person's response to stressors can vary. Roy[19] argues that this is controlled by three sets of stimuli:

- *focal*: those immediately present for the individual
- *contextual*: those occurring alongside the focal stimuli
- *residual*: those occurring from past learning and its effects.

As these three types of stimuli will never occur in exactly the same way each time, the response or adaptation will also vary. Consider the example of a patient who attends an outpatient clinic on two occasions for a wound dressing.

Visit 1

- The clinic is busy, many patients are waiting and the room is hot (contextual stimuli).
- The nurse attending the patient has had no lunch break, forgets his name and cannot remember what type of operation he has had (focal stimuli).
- On his last visit the wound was infected and the doctor applied a silver nitrate stick to some over-granulation; this was extremely painful (residual stimuli).

How do you think the patient coped with this visit?

Visit 2

- The clinic is quiet, cool and calm and the patient is asked to go straight in without waiting (contextual).
- A different nurse attends this week, who addresses him by his name, appears to know all about his wound and operation and explains the procedures. The wound is healthy with no complications (focal).

Now, although the patient's residual stimulus remains the same, both focal and contextual stimuli have changed. Would you expect the same behaviour on this visit?

Roy identified four principal adaptation systems that influence behaviour:

- *Physiological system*: the body's responses to food, fluids, oxygen, circulation, temperature, sensory input, exercise and rest.
- *Self-concept system*: the view that people hold of themselves, both physically and psychologically. It is concerned with how people see their own worth, both in their own eyes and in those of others.
- *Role mastery system*: focuses on the individual's need to have a place in society; the duties and responsibilities or rights and privileges they hold.
- *Interdependency system*: the balance between dependence and independence in relationships with others; levels of friendliness, dominance and competitiveness.

Nursing intervention will be required when there is a deficit or excess within one or more of these adaptation systems.

Assessment using Roy's model, as with other nursing models, consists of two stages. In the first stage the nurse will observe behaviour using each of the four adaptation systems as a framework. If there appears to be a problem of adaptation the nurse should move on to identify whether the factors creating this problem are focal, contextual or residual.

Planning must then identify the patient-centred goals in order of priority and the type of nursing intervention required to change either the stimuli or the patient adaptation level.

Nursing will generally concentrate on the focal stimuli as these will possibly be the primary cause of the patient's behaviour. However, this model is well suited to nurses experienced in behaviour modification and counselling techniques who have the confidence and capability to change adaptive behaviour caused by residual stimuli.

Roy's model has been used as the model of choice for patients nursed in a variety of settings, particularly in relation to changes in body image, e.g., lower extremity amputation.[20]

Roper's Activities of Living Model

Nancy Roper's original model[21] was the result of a research project undertaken between 1970 and 1974 and was a modification of previous work by Virginia Henderson published in 1966. Roper, Logan and Tierney were the first British nurses to use a

BOX 2.1 ACTIVITIES OF LIVING

1. Maintaining a safe environment
2. Communicating
3. Breathing
4. Eating and drinking
5. Eliminating
6. Personal cleansing and dressing
7. Controlling body temperature
8. Mobilizing
9. Working and playing
10. Expressing sexuality
11. Sleeping
12. Dying

From Roper N, Logan WW, Tierney AJ. *The Elements of Nursing*, 4th ed. Edinburgh: Churchill Livingstone; 1996.

conceptual model to form a basis of care. The focus of the model is 12 activities of living (Box 2.1); it acknowledges that all individuals are involved in activities that enable them to live. The model embraces the concept of an individual progressing along a continuum with varying degrees of dependence and independence, according to age and health. Movement can be in either direction and it should not be assumed that everyone can reach their full potential in all 12 activities. The key to using this model is the nurse's ability to assess the person's level of independence in each of the activities of living. Patient goals should be centred around the amount of nursing help required to move along the dependence/independence continuum.

For each activity of living listed in Box 2.1, the nurse should establish:

- what the patient can normally do
- what the patient can do now
- what the patient cannot do now
- what problems may develop.

The assessment should, where possible, involve both patient and nurse in the process of identifying actual and potential problems. Not all activities may be a cause of problems; the nurse should, as always, prioritize the goals of care.

Nursing intervention will follow three models of action, as identified by Roper:

- prevention strategies
- providing comfort (physical and mental)
- enabling the patient to seek help to take responsibility for self-care.

This model is widely used in nursing in the UK and has been criticized as following the medical model on the grounds that the activities of living are equivalent to physiological responses.

Interaction Models

Interaction models emphasize the social meanings people put upon all aspects of their life and the interpersonal relationships between individuals. This study of interaction between people originates from the theory of symbolic interactionism, which postulates that the importance of social life lies in providing the person with language, self-concept and role-taking ability.[22] The major focuses of such nursing models are therefore perception, communication, role and self-concept.[13] The key to using this type of model is to elicit the *patient's definition* of the situation; thus the model strongly identifies the active role an individual plays in any interaction.

These models are therefore unsuited to a philosophy of care that perpetuates the notion that the patient should be passive and the nurse active. Obviously in areas such as intensive care nursing, when the patient is unconscious, the nurse's active role is necessary. However, in many areas of wound care, interaction with patients is a central facet of management. The most widely used model from this school of thought is the Riehl (later to become Riehl-Sisca) interaction model.[12,23]

Riehl's Interaction Model

Riehl pays particular attention to psychological and sociological systems and underplays the importance of physiological systems as the primary focus of nursing problems. She believes that the essence of good assessment is when nurses attempt to 'enter the subjective world of patients'. It is only then that the nurse is able to help a patient adopt a more appropriate behaviour or role.

Nursing problems arise when there are disturbances within one or more of the three parameters – psychological, sociological or physiological.

Riehl does not give a particular assessment framework but suggests the use of the 'FANCAP' mnemonic – fluids, aeration, nutrition, communication, activity, pain. The FANCAP system was originally designed as a teaching tool and provides a bridge between nursing science and the patient.

In the first stage of assessment the nurse ascertains if the patient is adopting a role appropriate to the present situation. If there appears to be a disturbance in role, is it due to physiological, psychological or sociological parameters?

Patient-centred goals should then be identified and activities planned for patient and nurse. Nursing intervention will centre on role playing, thus extending the range of behaviour open to the patient and increasing the nurse's understanding of the patient's problem.

The interaction model offers an approach that is very different from system or developmental models. It has been used widely in psychiatric nursing, where the emphasis is on psychological and social problems. It is unlikely to find popularity in mainstream areas of wound management, but can be useful when caring for patients with factitious or self-inflicted wounds (see Chapter 6).

Planning Individualized Care

It is important when assessing the patient to consider the outcome or goal that is to be achieved. This is often the most difficult part of the problem-solving process, especially for the inexperienced nurse. Often goals are formulated around what the nurse is trying to achieve and not what the patient may want, and this disjuncture can form the basis of patients feeling disempowered in the care exchange.

SETTING GOALS AND OUTCOMES FOR PATIENTS WITH WOUNDS

It is essential that the aims of management are established following assessment, as without them care will lack direction and evaluation will be impossible. This is not to say that once goals have been set they can never be changed, as unforeseen events may necessitate their revision. For example, following an operation to remove her appendix, Miss Susan James, a 28-year-old secretary, wished to return to work within 2 weeks of the operation. Her plan of care stated this to be one of the goals. However, 7 days postoperatively she developed a wound infection which delayed healing and necessitated antibiotic therapy. Therefore, following evaluation of the case at 7 days it was necessary to formulate a new goal, taking into account the patient's general condition and that of the wound.

Although goal setting should be patient centred, in cases such as Susan's, the nurse's professional knowledge is required to advise the patient on what is the most reasonable and safest goal. Susan may still wish to return to her employment within the original goal of 14 days, but she should be advised that this may cause further complications of healing and result in delaying the final outcome of care – complete wound healing.

DISTINGUISHING GOALS FROM OUTCOMES

Goals and outcomes are terms that are often used interchangeably and can be confusing to students. There is no set rule as to which should be used as the definitions are similar[24]:

- *Goal*: an object of effort or ambition.
- *Outcome*: a result or visible effect.

Both refer to an end-point of care, both should be measurable and both should be evaluated against the level of care received.

It may be simpler to define them by saying that an overall outcome can be achieved by the setting of step-by-step goals. To use the analogy of a football match, the *outcome* of the match is whether a team wins, loses or draws. This outcome is dictated by the number of *goals* scored during the match. The outcome of care can be considered to be the ultimate aim of management. Whether or not it is achieved will depend on reaching step-by-step goals of care that the nurse and patient have set out for themselves.

SETTING OUTCOMES

Difficulty may be experienced when setting an outcome of management for patients with wounds because of the complexity of the wound healing process and the different types of wounds encountered.

Acute Wounds

For patients with acute wounds the outcome will normally be that of complete healing. Acute surgical wounds should heal within a predicted period without complication.

Therefore, when setting outcomes for a patient following this type of surgery, it is possible to be objective not only about the healing potential but also about the time in which healing should be achieved. This is a good marker for evaluation, as there should be a predictable decrease in wound size as the days to healing progress. Failure to correspond with this may indicate that all is not well with the wound healing process.

Although acute wounds may be easier to evaluate in terms of healing time, it should be remembered that healing is not always the desired outcome; the patient may have other motives and the nurse should be aware that if a wound is not healing as predicted and there are no obvious clinical signs to account for this delay, other factors should be considered.

Although difficult to prove, there is some evidence that a minority of acute wound cases include some degree of self-inflicted injury by patients who have an ulterior motive for prolonging the wound.

It is important to remember that complete healing should not be achieved at all costs, as the management and intervention used to achieve this may compromise the patient's quality of life.

Quality of life usually becomes more of an issue when dealing with patients whose wounds are longstanding and chronic.

Chronic Wounds

The outcome of care for patients with a chronic wound is more difficult to plan, as often healing will not be achieved for many months or years, if at all.

Chronic wounds are formed when predisposing conditions such as diabetes impair the tissue's ability to heal the damage. It is not unusual for individuals to have lived with a leg ulcer for 30 years or experienced an unhealed wound sinus for many months.

Malignant wounds will not be expected to heal and in most cases will become worse; therefore the outcome of care is palliation. The prime objective is alleviation of distressing symptoms, thereby maximizing the patient's quality of life. The principle, however, remains the same: whatever the stated outcome, it should be set against measurable and observable goals.

In palliative care settings the goal of care is guided by the WHO four cornerstones of care that focus on symptom control, teamwork, relationships and communication. The overarching aim is to provide quality of life. The domains of practice highlighted

---

Case Study 2.2

Venous Ulcer

....

Eleanor Banks has a venous ulcer on her right leg. She is currently having compression bandaging but the nurses would like her to complement this therapy with leg elevation.

The *outcome* of the care is to achieve complete healing of the ulcer within 4–5 months. It is necessary to formulate some patient-centred goals to achieve this. Look at the following goal: does it satisfy the three criteria outlined above?

Goal: Eleanor to elevate both legs at regular intervals during the day.

This goal does not really comply with the criteria as it gives no indication of 'how well' we want Eleanor to elevate her legs. The 'condition' under which she is to elevate them is not stated as she will not know how regular is regular! The only thing she knows is that it is to be achieved during the day. Only the 'patient response' is stated, which is that she is required to elevate her legs. No date is given as to when she is to achieve the goal by, therefore how will the nurses know when to evaluate if it is being achieved or not?

---

by EWMA[6] echo the WHO framework and the care of palliative wounds should be directed by the aspirations laid down by the institutional philosophy of the clinical environment and by best available evidence focusing on pain control and comfort.

SETTING GOALS

Patient goals should be defined by the following precise criteria:

- *How well*? The standard or degree of accuracy at which we expect the patient to perform.
- *Condition*: The circumstances under which the patient is to do it.
- *Patient response*: What is it we want the patient to be able to do?

It is not always easy to write clear criteria which are also measurable and observable as illustrated in Case study 2.2. It is best to avoid using subjective terms such as 'know', 'understand' and 'learn', as these do not tell us very much about how or what the patient is able to do.

Practice Points

How should this goal be written? Try to write it yourself before looking at the answer.

A more useful statement of the goal is as follows.

Goal: Eleanor to elevate both legs at height above heart level for one hour in the morning and one hour in the evening by 10 March.

The goal now defines the patient response (elevation), the conditions (1 hour twice a day) and how well? (at a height above heart level).

Although this goal states all the criteria, unless the nurse has fully explained why the patient must elevate her legs and the best way this can be achieved, this goal may seem rather daunting or the patient may not realize the importance elevation plays in the healing process.

As previously stated, goals must be patient centred and individualized. Eleanor needs to know that she can achieve this goal by lying on a sofa with her feet on the arm of the sofa; however, she may not own a sofa or may have a chest condition which prevents her from lying down. All these facts should have been ascertained during the assessment process so that this goal can be achieved by some other means.

It is still necessary to evaluate at the stated time whether Eleanor has been able to achieve her goal. If not, then changes to her care programme may be required.

Planning and writing outcomes and goals can be time-consuming and difficult. They are also dependent on the practitioner's experience in deciding what is achievable for an individual patient.

Summary

This chapter has outlined ways of using a nursing model when assessing patients with different wound aetiologies nursed in a variety of settings. Nursing models are used throughout the following chapters, demonstrating their practical application in the clinical setting.

Models are classified as:
- Developmental
  - Peplau's model[10]
  - Orem's model[11]
- Systems
  - Roy's adaptation model[18]
  - Roper, Logan and Tierney's activities of living model[9]
- Interaction
  - Riehl's interaction model[23]

FURTHER READING

Clark D. Religion, medicine and community in the early origins of St. Christopher Hospice. *J Palliat Med.* 2001;4(3):353–360.

Department of Health (DoH). *The Patient's Charter.* London: Department of Health; 1995.

REFERENCES

1. Francis R. *The Mid-Staffordshire NHS Foundation Trust Public Inquiry chaired by Robert Francis QC HC 947.* London: Report of the Mid-Staffordshire NHS Foundation Trust Public Inquiry; 2013. The Stationery Office.
2. Garner J. Some thoughts and responses to the Francis report. *Psychoanalysis Psychotherapy.* 2014;28(2):211–219.
3. McCrae N. Whither nursing models? The value of nursing theories in the context of evidence based practice and multi-disciplinary healthcare. *J Adv Nurs.* 2011;68(1):222–229.
4. Graham J. Nursing theory and clinical practice: How three nursing models can be incorporated into the care of patients with end stage kidney disease. *CANNT J.* 2006;16(4):28–31.
5. Haigh C. Editorial: Embracing the theory/practice gap. *J Clin Nurs.* 2008;18:1–2.
6. EWMA; 2019. Available at: https://ewma.org/.
7. International consensus. *Optimising Wellbeing in People Living with a Wound. An Expert Working Group Review.* London: Wounds International; 2012. Available at: http://www.woundsinternational.com.
8. Moore Z, Butcher G, Corbett LQ, et al. AAWC, AWMA, EWMA Position Paper: managing wounds as a team. *J Wound Care.* 2014;23(5 suppl):S1–S38. Available at: https://ewma.org/it/what-we-do/ewma-projects/managing-wounds-as-a-team/.
9. Roper N, Logan WW, Tierney AJ. *The Elements of Nursing.* 4th ed. Edinburgh: Churchill Livingstone; 1996.
10. Peplau H. *Interpersonal Relations in Nursing.* New York: G P Putnam; 1952.
11. Orem D. *Nursing – Concepts of Practice.* 5th ed. St Louis, Missouri: Mosby Yearbook; 1995.
12. Riehl JP, Roy C, eds. *Conceptual Models for Nursing Practice.* 2nd ed. New York: Appleton-Century-Crofts; 1980.
13. Fawcett J. *Analysis and Evaluation of Conceptual Models of Nursing.* 2nd ed. Philadelphia: F A Davies Company; 1989.
14. Maslow AH. *Motivation and Personality.* New York: Harper & Row; 1954.
15. Rogers ME. *Educational Revolution in Nursing.* New York: Macmillan; 1961.
16. Goodman B. *Psychology and Sociology in Nursing.* 2nd ed. London: Sage; 2015.
17. McKenna H, Pajnkihar M, Murphy F. *Fundamentals of Nursing Models, Theories and Practice.* 2nd ed. Oxford: Wiley-Blackwell; 2014.
18. Roy C, Andrews H. *The Roy Adaptation Model.* 2nd ed. Stamford, Connecticut: Appleton and Lange; 1999.
19. Roy C. Future of the Roy model: challenge to re-define adaptation. *Nurs Sci Q.* 1997;10(1):42–48.
20. Farsi Z, Azarmi S. Effect of Roy's adaption model-guided education on coping strategies of the veterans with lower extremity amputation: a double blind randomized controlled clinical trial. *Int J Community Based Nurs Midwifery.* 2016;4(2):127–136.
21. Roper N, Logan WW, Tierney AJ. *The Elements of Nursing.* Edinburgh: Churchill Livingstone; 1980.

22. Blumer H. *Symbolic Interactionism: Perspective and Method*. Englewood Cliffs, New Jersey: Prentice Hall; 1969.
23. Riehl-Sisca JP. The Riehl interaction model. In: Riehl-Sisca JP, ed. *Conceptual Models for Nursing Practice*. 3rd ed. Norwalk, Connecticut: Appleton and Lange; 1989.
24. *Concise Oxford Dictionary*. Oxford: Oxford University Press; 1982.

Riehl JP. The Riehl interaction model. In: Riehl JP, Roy C, eds. *Conceptual Models for Nursing Practice*. 2nd ed. New York: Appleton-Century-Crofts; 1980.
Roper N, Logan WW, Tierney AJ. *Using a Model for Nursing*. Edinburgh: Churchill Livingstone; 1983.

MCQS

1 *The deductive approach to knowledge emerged from:*
a. Psychology
b. Sociology
c. Law
d. Science

2 *Peplau was a nurse from:*
a. UK
b. France
c. Africa
d. USA

3 *Roper, Logan and Tierney's model focuses on:*
a. Activities of daily living
b. Self-adaption
c. Self-actualization
d. Mindfulness

INTERVENTION

Chapter 3

Principles of Wound Interventions

Samantha Holloway

Highlights

- Six decades on from the seminal work of George Winter, the evidence for the management of individuals with wounds still supports the use of moist wound healing
- Uncomplicated wounds healing by primary intention may only require a simple dressing for the first 48 hours, thereafter there is no requirement for the wound to be covered
- Principles of infection control to reduce the risk of wound complications include environmental hygiene measures, hand washing and an aseptic non-touch technique
- Wounds that are clean and appear to be healing may not require cleansing and should be left undisturbed to maintain an optimum environment for healing. Where cleansing is indicated, saline or water should be sufficient in the majority of cases
- Wound bed preparation and TIMERS still provide appropriate guiding principles for the assessment and management (including dressing choice) of an individual with a wound
- Medical devices and adjunctive therapies, in addition to dressings, are integral to the care of some individuals with specific wound aetiologies

Key Issues

This chapter introduces the reader to principles of wound interventions, including:
- wound healing by primary and secondary intention
- infection control
- wound bed preparation
- TIMERS
- devices and advanced interventions for management of wounds

Introduction

The range of interventions to manage individuals with wounds has increased exponentially over the last two decades. The potential armamentarium of options include dressings and topical agents, physical devices and biological substance; however, national and local policies may dictate the availability of such therapies. Although such technologies can make a major contribution to the management of wounds,[1] the principles of wound interventions such as maintaining a moist wound environment and eliminating dead or devitalized tissue from the wound bed, reducing the risk of infection are the cornerstone of wound management.

This chapter traces the history of wound treatments that have underpinned the development of today's wound therapies. It then focuses on the basic principles and techniques of wound interventions that should inform the clinical practice of all nurses involved in wound care.

Historical Perspective

In his 1975 book, Guido Majino examines the evolution of how wounds were treated through history.[2] Charting various interventions used across the world over time, this author perceptively states:

A million years ago, as now, a wound implied three major medical problems: mechanical disruption, bleeding and infection. Nature is prepared to cope with all three, but man [sic] can help, even with simple means.

EARLY HISTORY

For early humans most wounds and injuries were the result of accidents and fighting. These injuries represented a life-threatening problem, with blood loss being a major factor; haemostasis was achieved using whatever materials came readily to hand, including sand, leaves and faeces.

Records from early history that provide clues to common wounds include 25,000-year-old cave paintings in Spain, clay tablets from the Sumerians and papyrus from the Egyptians.[3] Surgery was performed in China, Egypt and Mesopotamia, and wound treatments included herbal medicines, sutures made from gum-coated linen, thorns and threads, resin, honey, lard, myrrh, milk and water.[4]

RECOGNIZING AND TREATING INFECTION

Hippocrates (460–377 BCE) encouraged suppuration to debride devitalized tissue and to reduce inflammation.[3] Nature, in Hippocrates' opinion, would heal wounds. Nearer to the time of Christ, Celsus (25 BCE–CE 50) wrote eight books on medicine and surgery. In *De medicina*, Celsus, for the first time, clearly described the four cardinal signs of infection, though these were not specifically describing wounds, '*Nota vera inflammationis sunt quattuor; rubor et tumor cum calor et dolor*' – the signs and symptoms of redness, swelling, heat and pain. Celsus also recommended the early closure of fresh wounds and the surgical debridement of contaminated wounds.[4]

Galen (CE 131–200) was a physician and anatomist who is thought to have produced over 500 books. His descriptions of routine wound management were typical of treatments of that time. Galen is famous for his theory of 'laudable pus', '*pus bonum et laudabile*', advocating that should a wound become infected and suppurate, this process should be allowed to continue.[4] He used dung, writing ink and wine as wound treatments and also made haemostatic concoctions out of frankincense and aloes mixed with eggs and fur clippings.[5] One of Galen's major contributions was to observe that spreading infection in a wound often resulted in widespread systemic sepsis and death.[6] However, Galen believed that when infection localized and then discharged itself, the wound would go on to heal without problems. During the Middle Ages medical practitioners misinterpreted this message to mean that pus formation was both desirable and necessary for healthy healing. Clean, uninfected wounds were inoculated with a variety of noxious substances in order to stimulate pus formation. These practices continued from the 7th to the 14th centuries. It was not until the 19th century that Pasteur and Lister managed to persuade their colleagues that mortality

rates could be reduced by using antiseptics and aseptic principles.[6]

Theodoric of Lucca (1205–1298) was most famous for his skills in inducing anaesthesia using mandrake- and opium-soaked sponges that were inhaled or swallowed. His contribution to wound care included his gentle approach to cleansing with honey and wine and dressing with lint soaked in warm wine.[5]

The anonymous Wellcome Manuscript 564 (dated 1392) gives a comprehensive account of wound care in London at this time. Naylor[7] reviewed its contents and reports definitions of acute wounds and chronic ulcers, malignant and infected wounds. Treatments including compression bandaging, moist wound dressings, occlusive dressings, a nutritious diet and wound cleansing are described in detail in this document. Naylor also found a list of factors that prolong healing, with bullet points that cited systemic disease, impaired blood supply and unsuitable wound treatment as examples.

Andreas Vesalius (1514–1564) achieved much before the age of 29, mainly his contribution to anatomy and physiology.[7] As with Theodoric of Lucca, he rejected the harsher treatments, using instead eggs and oil to dress wounds.

Sir Charles Bell (1774–1842) was recognized for his work during the battle of Waterloo (1815).[8] This was an era when advances were being made in surgical technique and the development of surgical instruments. On hearing of the devastation at the battle, Bell travelled to Belgium with his assistant to find 50,000 dead or injured men. Both sides had suffered terrible injuries and Bell operated on these men 'until his clothes were stiff with blood' and his arms so tired they were 'powerless with exertion of using the knife'. Bell and other surgeons corresponded with each other and, through these letters, it is possible to gain some understanding of the standard of surgery at this time. Surgical debridement was a widespread procedure, with devitalized bone and muscle excised. The control of haemorrhage was also undertaken by using ligatures and the range of surgical instruments was quite sophisticated. Many men died of their injuries through sepsis and also tetanus that, today, would be treatable.

Pasteur (1822–1895) discovered micro-organisms and bacteria, although initially his interest was not in patients with infection but in the role of bacteria in the fermentation of wines. Pasteur used his knowledge in this field to develop heat sterilization (pasteurization).[9]

Joseph Lister (1827–1912) became a professor of surgery in Glasgow in 1860. It was here that Lister worked on aseptic principles, antiseptic treatment of wounds and the use of carbolic spray during surgical procedures.[10] His interest was drawn to the problems related to sepsis and a high mortality rate amongst the patients in the Glasgow hospitals.

It was Lister who translated Pasteur's work to the field of patient care. Lister used Pasteur's findings to link suppuration of wounds with septicaemia, tetanus, gangrene and subsequent death. Although initially Lister used heat sterilization, he soon turned to chemical antiseptics. When Lister discovered how effective carbolic acid was, he was able to revolutionize surgical techniques. Infection and mortality rates fell dramatically as Lister used a combination of clean linen, a clean room, the use of carbolic acid spray and hand washing to reduce infection.[10]

THE ADOPTION OF ASEPTIC TECHNIQUES

The medical staff of the 19th century remained, for many years, unconvinced of the benefits of the principles advocated by Pasteur and Lister. It was only in 1876 when Lister published *On the antiseptic principle in the practice of surgery* that his profession took notice of him.[11] Gradually his work began to be expanded and developed, with steam sterilization used for surgical instruments and dressings. Theatre and dressing packs became available.

World War I

The introduction of aseptic technique during surgery and the use of the operating theatre (as opposed to the kitchen table) brought a more controlled environment to surgery. Scrubbing-up procedures, gloves and sterile dressings were other methods being developed to reduce wound infection. Tulle gras dressings were developed as a low-adherent dressing. Carbolic acid was found to have too many side effects[12] so Eusol[13] and Dakin's solution[14] became popular. Eusol (an acronym for Edinburgh University solution of lime) contained chlorinated lime and boric acid diluted with water. Dakin's solution contained chlorinated lime, boric acid and sodium carbonate. Infection was a real problem in World War

I, with contamination of wounds by earth and dirt being widespread, leading to gas gangrene and many subsequent deaths.[3]

ANTIBIOTICS

The first sulphonamide, prontosil rubrum, was developed in 1936 by Domagh (1895–1964) and its use transformed the prognosis of many bacterial diseases.[15] However, it had severe side effects on the kidneys and blood. By comparison, a virtually harmless antibiotic was soon to be discovered. Through his accidental discovery of penicillin, Fleming (1881–1955) revolutionized the care of many patients with infections. He found that bactericidal substances were released from *Penicillium* mould.[16] This finding was used in the treatment of humans with infection by Howard Florey and Ernst Chain in 1941.

At the same time that Fleming was working on penicillin, Colebrook was studying the role of haemolytic *Streptococcus* in relation to childbirth and the problems of puerperal sepsis. Colebrook discovered that sulphonamide contained in the dye prontosil was active against streptococcal infection. Subsequently Colebrook looked at the problem of streptococcal infection in burn patients. Using asepsis and antiseptics, topical penicillin cream and stringent cross-infection measures, he much improved the prognosis for burns victims.[17] Due to his political activities, the 1952 Fireguard Act was introduced as a way of preventing burns.[18]

DRESSINGS AND WOUND CLEANSING

Around 2500 BC clay tablets in Mesopotamia recorded the use of milk and water to cleanse wounds and the application of honey or resin dressings or myrrh and frankincense.[19] Hippocrates (460–377 BCE) advocated early haemostasis and the treatment of contused wounds with salves. Many years later, a French surgeon, de Mondeville (1260–1320), also used water to cleanse wounds. He recommended compress dressings of hot wine, encouraging patients to rest and eat nutritious food.[5] However, there were many differences in treatments. In de Mondeville's time, another surgeon, de Chauliac (1300–1368), was using oily salves and mesh packing to promote pus formation.

Paracelsus (1493–1541) developed a theory that man had a juice that continually circulated around the body to keep the tissues and organs healthy and in a good state of repair. Consequently he recommended that all medicines, treatments and dressings should aim to maintain these body juices in the optimum condition. To this end he opposed the use of boiling oil on wounds.[20]

Ambroise Paré (1510–1593) was the founder of military surgery in the 16th century.[21] An advocate of the 'laudable pus' theory, his decision to stop using noxious substances to induce infection came about when the boiling oil he was using on the battlefield ran out and he used, as an alternative, egg yolks on the battle wounds of soldiers.[22] Compared with soldiers treated with boiling oil, soldiers treated with egg yolk had a higher survival rate and Paré changed his philosophy. Subsequently, Paré said, 'I dressed his wounds, God healed him', the quote for which he is famous: '*Je le pansay, et Dieu le guarit*'. He used powder of rock alum, verdigris, Roman vitriol, rose honey and vinegar boiled together to form a wound dressing.[5] Although German, Heister (1683–1758) was most influential in France. He described wound treatments, especially the bandages and dressings that were used. He carefully catalogued wounds in great detail, describing their size and shape, and the cocktails of dressings that were used.[5]

Joseph Gamgee (1828–1886) qualified first as a veterinary surgeon and later studied medicine. He gained experience in the Crimean War and at the Royal Free Hospital in London, going on to work in Birmingham. It was here that Gamgee became interested in wound healing. He wrote of the need for 'utmost gentleness in dealing with wounds and infrequent changes of dressing'.[23] Through working with cotton wool and gauze, he designed an 'absorbent and antiseptic surgical dressing'. This consisted of pads of degreased cotton wool covered in gauze that was bleached to give it absorbency. In these early days this dressing formed a barrier to cross-infection and provided a warm environment at the wound bed. Gamgee also soaked his dressing in phenol and iodine occasionally.[24]

The Development of Moist Wound Healing

The zoologist George Winter (1927–1981) investigated wound healing in cutaneous wounds in the domestic pig. He later became interested in wound dressings and worked on covering wounds in an experimental model (using the pig) and observing healing rates. In his most famous piece of work, Winter observed that wounds covered with an occlusive dressing healed faster than those left to dry out.[25] It was from this work that the principles of moist wound healing were developed. Research in human wounds[26,27] confirmed a similar acceleration in healing under moist conditions.

Under dry conditions the bed of an open wound rapidly dries out and forms a scab made up of dead and dying cells. New epidermal cells migrate in the moist environment found under the scab, so extending the healing phase. In a moist environment exudate bathes the wound bed with nutrients and many modern dressing materials are designed to maintain moisture.

Prominent pharmacists including Turner[28] and Thomas[29] have described the functions of an ideal dressing. These criteria are brought together to define the essential characteristics of a dressing[30]:

- non-adherent
- impermeable to bacteria
- capable of maintaining a high humidity at the wound site while removing excess exudate
- thermally insulating
- non-toxic and non-allergenic
- comfortable and conformable
- capable of protecting the wound from further trauma
- requires infrequent dressing changes
- cost-effective
- long shelf life
- available both in hospital and in the community.

Subsequently Thomas and Leigh[31] concluded that the optimal conditions for wound healing are:

- moist with exudate but not macerated
- free of clinical infection and excessive slough
- free of toxic chemical particles or fibres released by the dressing
- at the optimum temperature
- undisturbed by frequent or unnecessary dressing changes
- at the correct pH.

Current clinical practice continues to uphold the principles of moist wound healing,[32] which have been incorporated into the principles of wound bed preparation[33] and the TIME acronym[34,35] (tissue, infection, moisture, edge), which can be very useful in guiding wound assessment.[36] The principles of TIME have been extended to TIMERS, which takes into account the importance of repair and regeneration as well as social factors.[37]

The range of modern wound dressings is outlined in Table 3.1, which lists their properties, presentation, dressing change frequency and indications.

Interventions for Wound Healing by Primary Intention

Wound healing by primary intention (Fig. 3.1) describes where the wound edges are apposed, that is brought together by sutures, staples, glue or Steri-Strips. Here wound healing occurs mainly by connective tissue formation. Delayed primary closure is used where there may be a risk of contamination or infection, for example if the patient has undergone emergency abdominal surgery with associated faecal spillage. In this instance, some of the layers of tissue are closed, and the sutures are placed in readiness for the remainder of the wound to be closed after 48 hours when the risk of infection has lessened.[38]

The vast majority of closed wounds heal without any complications. However the biggest risk is surgical site infection (SSI)[39] (Fig. 3.2). Existing evidence from the National Institute of Health and Clinical Excellence (NICE) indicates that SSI accounts for up to 16% of all healthcare-associated infections (HCAIs).[40] Procedures that carry a lower risk of infection are those in orthopaedics (<1%), with large bowel surgery being higher at >10%. As many SSIs develop after discharge from hospital, it is important that the patient and their carers are provided with information and advice about recognizing wound healing problems at an early stage in order to seek out prompt treatment.[40]

For uncomplicated closed wounds a simple dressing is suggested.[41] This may be a semipermeable film dressing which helps to control the levels of moisture and facilitates wound assessment more easily. However patient preference may dictate an absorbent dressing where the wound is less visible. Such dressings have some permeability characteristics and so facilitate evaporation of moisture and prevent maceration.

An early study by Chrintz et al. examining the need for a wound dressing on clean and clean-contaminated surgical wounds indicated that following haemostasis, where the wound is sealed by fibrin this should afford sufficient protection from moisture and bacterial contamination after 24 hours without the need for dressing.[42] More recently, evidence to support early or delayed removal of dressings on clean and clean-contaminated surgical wounds has not highlighted any differences in terms complications.[43] This means that the choice of whether to use a dressing or not is often based on surgeon and/or patient preference.

When a postoperative dressing is used, some key principles for consideration include the following:

- Allow for limb or joint movement to reduce the risk of traction blistering.[41]
- Dressings applied in theatre need not be changed or disturbed unless there is a good reason for doing so, such as:
  - strike-through on the dressing as this is an increased risk for infection
  - the patient develops signs of local/spreading infection.

A summary of current recommendations for surgical wounds in the postoperative phase (defined as 3–5 days) is shown in Box 3.1.[44]

Interventions for Wound Healing by Secondary Intention

INFECTION PREVENTION AND CONTROL

Hospital Environment

Existing international guidelines for the prevention of wound infection related to the physical hospital environment are available (Table 3.2).[45–47]

Hand Hygiene

The most effective method of preventing cross-infection is to use a good hand-washing technique. This is the cornerstone of the prevention of the spread of infection. As with the rest of the skin, hands carry bacteria that are permanently resident and which can only be eradicated for a few hours.[48] However, the skin can also be contaminated with transient pathogenic organisms, especially when hands are wet, rings are worn and skin is damaged.

TABLE 3.1   Range of Wound Dressings[a]

Dressing	Properties	Availability	Dressing Change	Indications
Absorbent	Often referred to as 'simple' dressings. Generally non-occlusive, permeable dressings which may be soft viscose, polyester-bonded. Some may also be 'super-absorbers'	Sheets of various sizes from 5 × 5 cm and as a rope dressing	Designed to stay in place for several days. Should be changed when leakage is imminent	Primary or secondary dressing. Lightly exuding wounds. Some have a waterproof outer covering so allow showering/bathing
Films	Polyurethane or co-polymer with a semipermeable adhesive layer. Conformable. Clear dressing allows wound inspection	Sheets ranging from 5 × 5 cm to large theatre drapes	Designed to stay in place for several days. Should be changed when leakage is imminent	Primary or secondary dressing. Superficial and epithelializing wounds: minor burns, category 2 pressure ulcers. Postoperative dressing for sutured wounds, intravenous line sites
Wound contact layers	Low adherence to wound bed. Allow passage of exudate through dressing	Sheets of various sizes from 5 × 5 cm	Designed to stay in place for several days. Supplementary absorbent padding can be changed more frequently without disturbing wound bed	Primary dressing. Contact layer that can be used with absorbent padding
Antimicrobial, i.e., silver, iodine, PHMB, chlorohexidine, DACC	Donates antimicrobial agent from dressing to wound bed. Controls bacterial burden. Effective against a broad spectrum of micro-organisms	Variety of wound dressings – sheets and cavity dressings	When saturated, leaking or when active agent has been absorbed	Where micro-organisms are adversely affecting healing. Clinical signs of infection. Primary dressings. All wound types
Alginates	Highly absorbent. Low adherent as gels on contact with exudate. Some have haemostatic properties	Sheets of various sizes, packing and ropes	Designed to stay in place for several days. Change when saturated or leaking imminent	Moderately to heavily exuding wounds of all aetiologies. Flat and cavity wounds, sinus tracts
Protease modulators	Mixture of collagen and oxidized regenerated cellulose. Donates collagen to wound bed to stimulate cellular migration and new tissue development. Non-adherent and absorbent	Sheets of various sizes	Designed to be used on debrided wounds or those where no debris is present. Wounds should be free of the clinical signs of infection. Usually require a secondary dressing	Full-thickness pressure ulcers, venous leg ulcers and mixed aetiology leg ulcers that do not show signs of healing. Also available with added silver to manage bioburden

TABLE 3.1   Range of Wound Dressings[a]—cont'd

Dressing	Properties	Availability	Dressing Change	Indications
Foams	Absorbent, conformable. Atraumatic at dressing change. Easy to apply and remove	Sheets of various sizes. Cavity dressings. Some are adhesive. Some are shaped	Designed to stay in place for several days. Change when saturated or leaking imminent	Moderately to heavily exuding wounds of all aetiologies
Hydrocolloids	Absorbent. Hydrophilic colloid particles bound to polyurethane foam. Impermeable to bacteria. Some are semi-clear	Sheets of various sizes and shapes. Usually adhesive. Various thicknesses	Designed to stay in place for several days. Change when saturated or leaking imminent	Low to moderately exuding wounds of all aetiologies. Flat and cavity wounds
Hydrogels	Rehydrate the wound bed by donating water. Used to facilitate autolysis where necrotic or devitalized tissue is present. Non-adherent. Water or glycerine based, crossed-linked polymer that contains 80–99% water	Sachets or tubes of gel, sheets or strips	Usually require a secondary dressing to hold gel in place and to prevent evaporation of water. Can be left for several days but can macerate surrounding skin if not changed frequently enough. Change when leaking imminent	Dry wound beds of all aetiologies. Caution where gangrene might be mistaken for necrotic tissue (check vascular status). Not recommended for heavily exuding wounds
Odour control	Absorb toxins and adsorb odour. Majority contain charcoal which acts as a filter. Many dressings are composite in nature and include absorbent layers of alginate and/or foam to manage exudate	Sheets of various sizes, gels	Change when saturated or leaking imminent. Gels will require a secondary dressing	Fungating and other malodourous wounds
Medicinal honey	Antibacterial, anti-inflammatory, debriding, deodorizing and stimulating of tissue growth	Available in sheets of various sizes and ointments	May require daily dressing change if wound infected	Infected wounds, acute and chronic, oncology-related lesions and burns. Check for allergies to bee pollen or products. Can cause maceration so protect surrounding skin

[a]For further information refer to Cowan T, ed. *The Wound Care Handbook 2018–19*. 11th ed. Salisbury, UK: MA Healthcare. Available at https://www.woundcarehandbook.com/

DACC, Dialkylcarbamoyl chloride; PHMB, polyhexamethylene biguanide.

The WHO infection prevention campaign,[49] known as *My 5 Moments for Hand Hygiene* (Fig. 3.3), best summarises the crucial times healthcare professionals should perform hand hygiene:

- before touching a patient
- before clean/aseptic procedures
- after body fluid exposure/risk
- after touching a patient
- after touching patient surroundings.

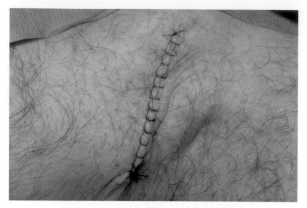

Fig. 3.1 Wound healing by primary intention.

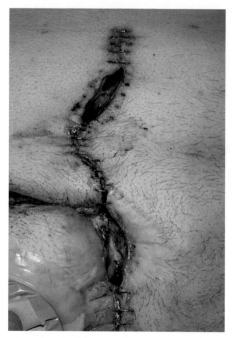

Fig. 3.2 Dehisced abdominal wound due to surgical site infection.

BOX 3.1 RECOMMENDATIONS FOR POSTOPERATIVE SURGICAL WOUNDS

- Use an aseptic, non-touch technique for changing and removing dressings.
- Keep the frequency of dressing changes to a minimum to avoid disrupting healing tissue.
- Use sterile saline for wound cleansing up to 48 hours after surgery.
- Use tap water for wound cleansing after 48 hours if the wound has separated or has been surgically opened to drain pus. Antiseptic agents are considered unnecessary for general wound cleansing but may be of value when irrigating an infected cavity wound.
- Where periwound skin maceration occurs or is considered to be a risk (e.g., if an enteral fistula is present or if there are excessive exudate levels) consider skin barrier products.
- Use an interactive dressing (i.e., one that promotes the wound healing process through the creation and maintenance of a local, warm, moist environment underneath the chosen dressing) for surgical wounds that are healing by secondary intention.[37] The dressing should be left in place for as long as indicated. A continual assessment process ensures dressing changes are kept to a minimum.
- Advise patients that they can shower safely 48 hours after surgery.
- Do not use topical antimicrobial agents for surgical wounds that are healing by primary intention.
- Refer the patient to wound care specialists if required for advice on appropriate dressings and care.
- Educate patients and carers and other healthcare professionals on optimal wound care, how to identify a wound that is failing to heal and who to contact if they are concerned about a possible SSI.[37]

From Milne J, Vowden P, Fumarola S, Leaper D. Postoperative incision management made easy. *Wounds UK.* 2012; suppl 8(4). Available from www.wounds-uk.com/made-easy, with permission.

Aseptic Technique

There are fundamental principles that need to be adhered to when undertaking wound care procedures. The most important of these relates to carrying out an aseptic technique to prevent HCAI. Fig. 3.4 shows information posters to highlight when an aseptic technique should be used. It refers to the Aseptic Non-Touch Technique (ANTT®), an international campaign originally proposed in 2001.[50] Box 3.2 summarizes the types of ANTT.[51] Please refer to your own local policies and procedures for aseptic technique.

Application of basic principles such as the use of gloves, hand washing, wound irrigation and sterile dressings can be adapted to a range of situations, from the hospital patient in a surgical ward with an acute wound and to the patient nursed at home with chronic leg ulcers. Wearing gloves should never replace scrupulous hand washing but is an essential precaution when the skin is broken, as transmission of blood-borne viruses is possible through damaged skin.

Publishing Body/Guideline	Country	Year of Publication
NICE: Infection prevention and control[a]	United Kingdom	2014
ECDC: Organisation of infection prevention and control in healthcare settings[b]	European Union	2015
WHO: Guidelines on core components of infection prevention and control programmes at the national and acute health care facility level[c]	Global/international	2016

TABLE 3.2 Infection Control Guidelines for the Hospital Environment

[a]National Institute for Health and Care Excellence. *Infection prevention and control*. London: NICE; 2014. Available at: https://www.nice.org.uk/guidance/qs61

[b]European Centre for Disease Prevention and Control. *Organisation of infection prevention and control in healthcare settings*. Solna: ECDC; 2015. Available at: https://ecdc.europa.eu/en/publications-data/directory-guidance-prevention-and-control/measures-in-hospitals

[c]World Health Organization. *Guidelines on core components of infection prevention and control programmes at the national and acute health care facility level*. Geneva: WHO; 2016. Available at: https://www.who.int/gpsc/ipc-components/en/

When managing patients with chronic wounds, maintaining hygiene is important; therefore, appropriate methods to keep the wound and patient clean should be considered. Soaking the lower limb in a bucket of tap water with an emollient (where appropriate) will help to cleanse the wound and the surrounding skin and can offer a psychological benefit. Generally showering is preferable to bathing as it is more hygienic, but can be difficult for frail, elderly patients. Nurses need to use their clinical judgement and take into account environmental factors in determining the best approach.

Wound Cleansing

Despite the lack of evidence, routine cleansing of wounds is still practised in many areas of wound care.[52] Indications for cleansing are clear if the underlying principles of wound healing and bacterial colonization are understood.

It is often believed that the presence of bacteria on a wound bed is harmful and that wound cleansing will eliminate bacteria, so promoting a healthy wound bed and healing. However, research has demonstrated that most granulating wound bed surfaces are colonized with bacteria and that these do not often cause a problem or delay in healing.[53] Indeed, normal wound repair requires the bactericidal activity and growth factors present in the inflammatory exudate.[54] Removal of wound fluid through cleansing and then drying of the wound may only deplete the healing tissue of these vital components and contradicts the principles of moist wound healing.[52]

It is not possible or even advisable[55] to remove all bacteria from the wound surface. However management of bioburden and biofilm needs to be considered when making a clinical judgement regarding cleaning a wound.

Wounds should only be cleansed to remove excess exudate, slough or necrotic tissue and remnants of old dressing material, all of which can become a focus for infection.[52] However, wounds caused by accidental trauma often contain large amounts of debris and are grossly contaminated and these require thorough cleansing.[56] Patients with burns and thermal injuries also require wound cleansing, initially as a first aid measure to reduce the extent of the injury but also because the wound is at greater risk of infection.[57]

TYPES OF CLEANSING SOLUTION

The use of antiseptic cleansing agents is rarely indicated in routine wound cleansing[58] because the required mechanical cleansing to remove excess debris can be safely achieved using water or saline. In addition, existing research has demonstrated that some antiseptic wound cleansing agents can damage healthy wound cells, inhibiting their viability and phagocytic activity.[59] Several studies have shown the effectiveness of normal saline, tap water, distilled water, boiled water and antibacterial solutions in not only in lowering bacterial counts but also in reducing infection, although no differences have been detected between these solutions.[60]

Whilst acknowledging that antiseptics may have a detrimental effect on healing, it is also accepted that the consequences of increased bioburden, biofilm and infection mean that use of saline or tap water

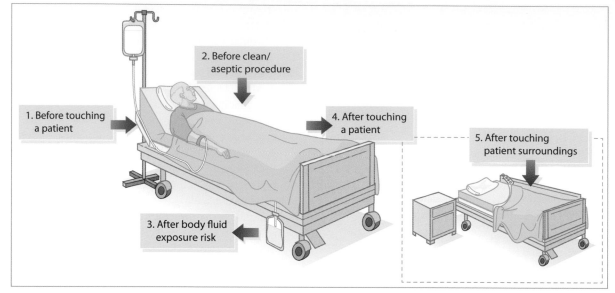

Fig. 3.3 My 5 Moments for Hand Hygiene. (From Sax H, Allegranzi B, Uçkay I, Larson E, Boyce J, Pittet D. 'My five moments for hand hygiene': a user-centred design approach to understand, train, monitor and report hand hygiene. *J Hosp Infect* 2007;67(1):9–21, with permission of WHO.)

may not be sufficient. Therefore there is a role for antiseptics such as antiseptic wound irrigation fluids and gels for cleansing,[52] which include iodine in various forms (povidone-iodine and cadexomer iodine), chlorhexidine, silver and polyhexamethylene biguanide. Roberts et al.[61] highlight the important contribution that topically applied antiseptics can make in conjunction with or as an alternative to systemic antibiotics in wound care, particularly in the era of antimicrobial stewardship. Therefore this is another example of the need for exercising clinical judgement in decision making.

METHOD OF CLEANSING

Swabbing a wound with cotton wool or gauze is inadvisable and largely ineffective as these can shed fibres. Instead the use of a non-woven gauze swab and a gloved hand is preferable.[52] Where large amounts of fluid are required to remove debris, this is best achieved by wound irrigation. Gentle irrigation for normal cleansing can be achieved with the use of a syringe (no needle) or quill or a jug of warmed saline. When water is used, immersing the wound area in a bowl or bath may be an easy way to remove debris or exudate and may be less painful to

the patient. Careful consideration should be given to proper cleaning of equipment to maintain adequate infection control.

Other mechanical methods of cleansing include high-pressure, pulsatile irrigation devices, but these can expensive, require specialist training and are not widely used in general clinical practice.

An alternative approach is the use of a monofilament fibre pad, which is generally thought of as a method of debridement. However its use can help to get rid of superficial slough from the wound bed as well as dead tissue at the wound edge and periwound area.[52]

CONCLUSION

Cleansing of a wound should only be performed when clearly indicated and irrigation with saline or water should be sufficient in most cases. Wounds that are clean and appear to be healing may not require cleansing and should be left undisturbed to maintain an optimum environment for healing. However if wound healing appears to be delayed, consider the impact that bioburden and/or biofilm may be having and think about whether cleaning, use of antiseptic solution and/or debridement may be needed.

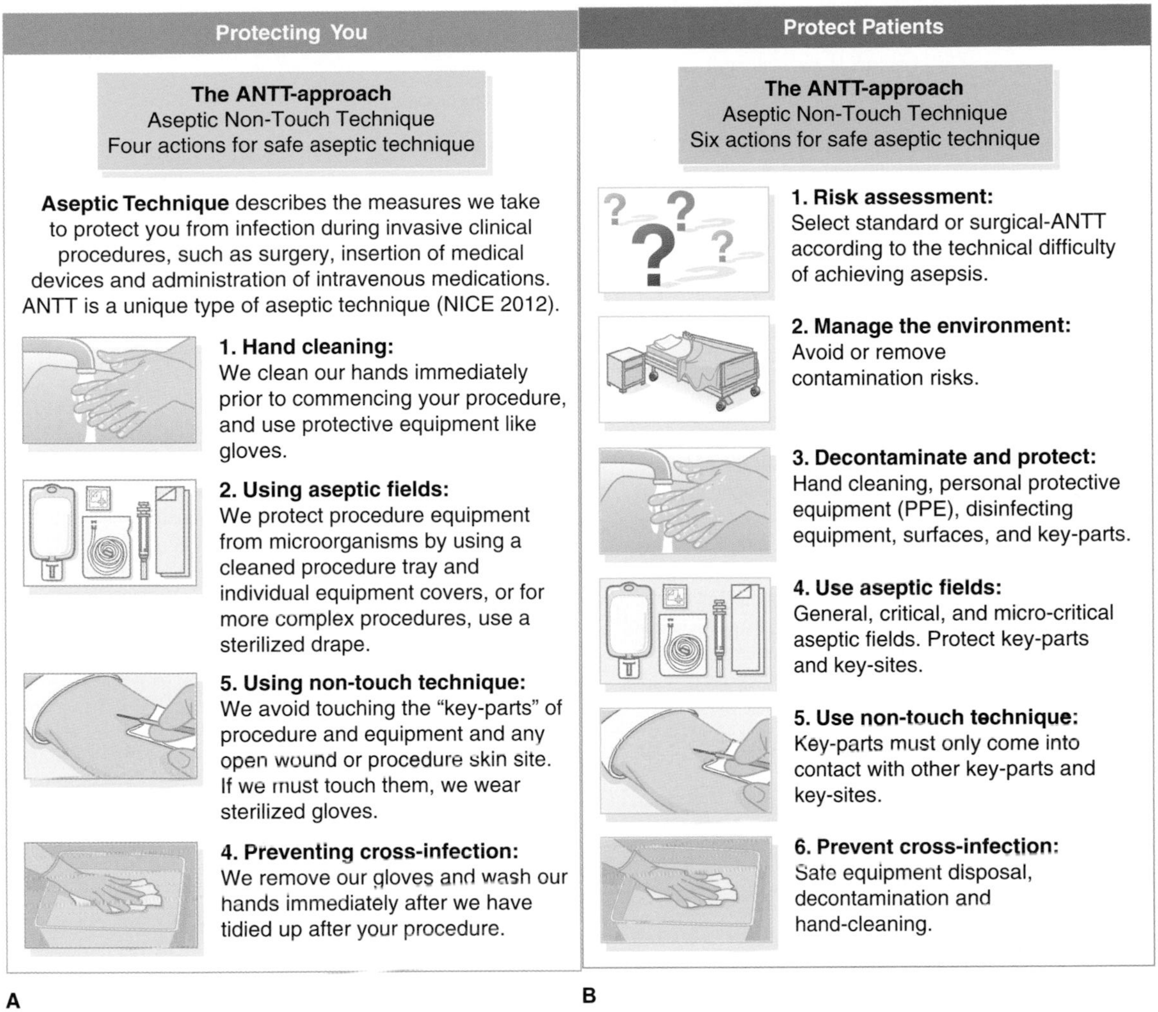

Protecting You	Protect Patients
The ANTT-approach Aseptic Non-Touch Technique Four actions for safe aseptic technique	**The ANTT-approach** Aseptic Non-Touch Technique Six actions for safe aseptic technique

Protecting You

Aseptic Technique describes the measures we take to protect you from infection during invasive clinical procedures, such as surgery, insertion of medical devices and administration of intravenous medications. ANTT is a unique type of aseptic technique (NICE 2012).

1. Hand cleaning:
We clean our hands immediately prior to commencing your procedure, and use protective equipment like gloves.

2. Using aseptic fields:
We protect procedure equipment from microorganisms by using a cleaned procedure tray and individual equipment covers, or for more complex procedures, use a sterilized drape.

5. Using non-touch technique:
We avoid touching the "key-parts" of procedure and equipment and any open wound or procedure skin site. If we must touch them, we wear sterilized gloves.

4. Preventing cross-infection:
We remove our gloves and wash our hands immediately after we have tidied up after your procedure.

Protect Patients

1. Risk assessment:
Select standard or surgical-ANTT according to the technical difficulty of achieving asepsis.

2. Manage the environment:
Avoid or remove contamination risks.

3. Decontaminate and protect:
Hand cleaning, personal protective equipment (PPE), disinfecting equipment, surfaces, and key-parts.

4. Use aseptic fields:
General, critical, and micro-critical aseptic fields. Protect key-parts and key-sites.

5. Use non-touch technique:
Key-parts must only come into contact with other key-parts and key-sites.

6. Prevent cross-infection:
Safe equipment disposal, decontamination and hand-cleaning.

A   B

Fig. 3.4 Aseptic Non-Touch Technique procedure. (A) Poster aimed at patients and (B) poster aimed at staff. (With permission from ANTT/Association for Safe Aseptic Practice.)

Assessment of Tissue Type

Wound healing by secondary intention (Fig. 3.5) describes a situation where the wound is left open to heal, i.e., a wound that was sutured that subsequently dehisced. Secondary intention also describes the majority of chronic wounds, i.e., leg ulcers, pressure ulcers and diabetic ulcers. Such wounds heal by the formation of granulation tissue and wound contraction. A review by Vermeulen at al. in 2005[62] was able to determine the superiority of one dressing over another for postoperative wounds healing by secondary intention. Therefore the choice of dressing should be based on an assessment of the wound bed and goal of treatment.

Guiding principles for interventions should take into account:

- a comprehensive assessment of the patient to include: history, examination, investigations, diagnosis and indicators of healing (HEIDI)[63] (Fig. 3.6)
- type of tissue type present in the wound bed (TIMERS[33–35]) (Fig. 3.7), i.e., necrotic, sloughy, infected, granulating, epithelializing, hypergranulation

BOX 3.2 TYPES OF ANTT®

There are two types of ANTT (surgical and standard) determined by a simple ANTT risk assessment.

- Standard-ANTT is used for procedures for which it is technically simple to achieve asepsis. Typically such a procedure will be of short duration and involve few small key-parts and key-sites. In standard-ANTT, key-parts are protected primarily by non-touch technique and individual micro-critical aseptic fields.
- Surgical-ANTT is required for procedures for which it is technically complex to achieve asepsis. These are of longer duration, involve large open sites and large or numerous key-parts. In contrast to standard-ANTT, in surgical-ANTT, key-parts are managed on one main critical aseptic field (sterile drape) and sterile gloves are essential.
- Aseptic fields in ANTT: The type of aseptic field and how it is managed is dependent upon the type of ANTT being utilized. ANTT uses three types of aseptic field: (a) critical aseptic field: a large sterile drape that is managed 'critically'; (b) micro-critical aseptic field: sterilized caps and covers etc. including the inside of some equipment packaging; (c) general aseptic field: a disinfected plastic tray, suitable-sized single-use cardboard tray. NB: general aseptic fields are not relied upon to maintain asepsis. They are used to promote asepsis whilst key-parts within them are protected by micro-critical aseptic fields.

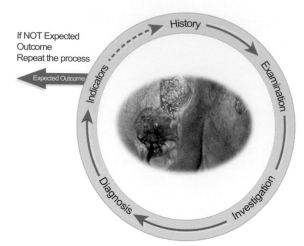

Fig. 3.6 HEIDI, a mnemonic for: history, examination, investigation, diagnosis and indicators of healing; a wound assessment concept developed by Keith Harding. (From Heinrichs EL, Llewellyn M, Harding K. Assessment of a patient with a wound. In: Gray D, Cooper P eds. *Wound Healing: A Systematic Approach to Advanced Wound Healing and Management.* 2005:1–27, with permission.)

- condition of the surrounding skin
- any known sensitivities or allergies to dressings or contact material.

HEALTHY GRANULATING AND EPITHELIALIZING WOUNDS

The aim of intervention for wounds that are in the proliferative phase of healing and producing granulation tissue is to maintain an environment conducive to healing. Following assessment of the patient, the wound characteristics and the social environment of the patient, a nursing model can be selected and a wound care plan formulated.

MOISTURE BALANCE

Although exudate is produced by all healthy open wounds, excessive exudate may be produced by particularly large wounds or deep cavities. If exudate is not controlled, leakage may occur which soils and stains clothes and bed clothes, causing discomfort and embarrassment. Excessive exudate can cause damage to the skin and maceration of the wound bed (Fig. 3.8) via enzymatic activity, in particular matrix metalloproteinases.[65] Exudate can be controlled by using absorbent dressing materials, by frequent dressing changes or by using a barrier

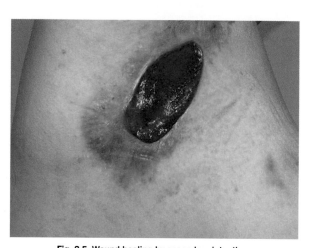

Fig. 3.5 Wound healing by secondary intention.

- need for debridement, which may be required on more than one occasion ('maintenance debridement'[64])
- moisture balance and level and type of exudate
- depth of the wound and presence of undermining or tunnelling

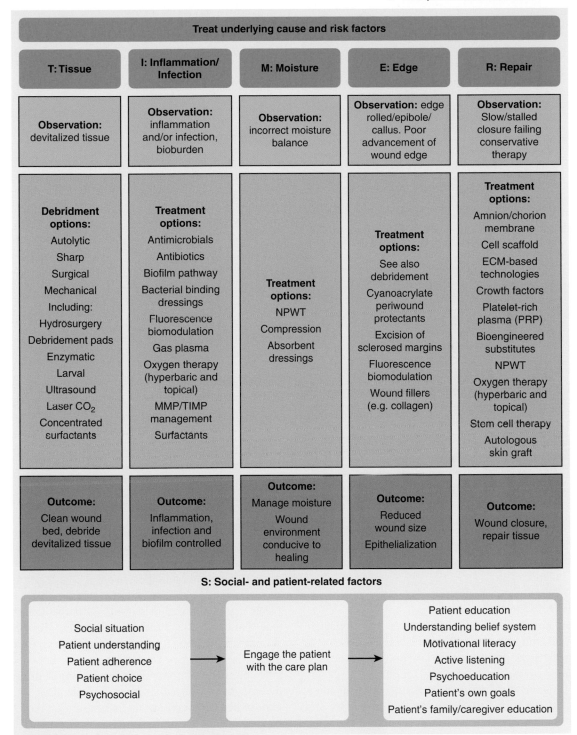

Fig. 3.7 TIMERS framework for hard-to-heal wounds. ECM, Extracellular matrix; MMP, matrix metalloproteinases; NPWT, negative-pressure wound therapy; TIMP, tissue inhibitors of metalloproteinases. (From Atkin L , Bućko Z, Conde Montero E, et al. Implementing TIMERS: the race against hard-to-heal wounds *J Wound Care*. 2019;1;23(Suppl 3a):S1–S50, with permission.)

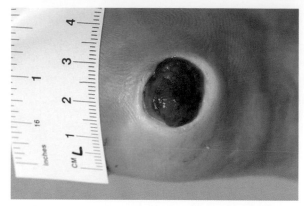

Fig. 3.8 Heel pressure ulcer showing periwound maceration.

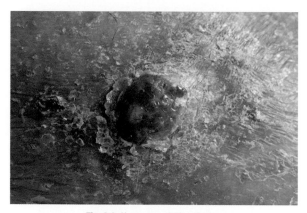

Fig. 3.9 Hypergranulation tissue.

cream.[66] The key to effective wound management is managing excess exudate and maintaining a moisture balance.

HYPERGRANULATION

Granulation tissue can be produced in excessive amounts and rise above the level of the skin. This is referred to as hypergranulation or overgranulation within a wound bed[67] (Fig. 3.9). Epithelial cells will only migrate over a flat surface; therefore an intervention is required to flatten the wound surface and thus facilitate re-epithelialization. Vuolo[67] proposed a framework for the management of hypergranulation which summarizes the likely cause and suggested management options (Fig. 3.10).

The application of silver nitrate sticks to cauterize the tissue is also used; however this is cautioned against as it can be painful for the patient.[67] In the absence of definitive evidence for the optimum approach, the use of permeable foam or film with a moderate level of pressure to inhibit further growth is recommended.

WOUND DEBRIDEMENT

The presence of sloughy, necrotic, devitalized tissue on the wound bed can delay healing and also increases the risk of wound infection (Fig. 3.11). It is important to remove devitalized tissue as quickly and efficiently as possible to reduce the bioburden of the wound and to control or prevent infection.[66] This can be difficult to achieve, however, as both slough and necrotic tissue are firmly stuck to the wound bed and cannot simply be wiped away. Methods of achieving wound debridement[68] are numerous and include surgical, sharp, autolytic, biosurgical (maggots), mechanical (i.e., use of monofilament pad, hydrosurgery, ultrasound) and chemical/enzymatic.

Surgical Debridement

This generally describes the removal of dead, necrotic/slough tissue at the time of an operation or during a subsequent re-exploration of a wound. It is the most direct form of debridement as it uses sharp instruments to remove the devitalized tissue[69] and is sometimes referred to as sharp surgical debridement.[70]

Sharp Debridement

Sharp debridement is by far the quickest and most effective method, as debridement is immediate and a healthy wound bed can result (Fig. 3.12). Here the devitalized or dead tissue is cut away from the healthy tissue using a scalpel or scissors at the patient's bedside. However, the clinician undertaking this procedure must be able to differentiate between healthy and unhealthy tissue and must also be knowledgeable about the anatomy of the area being debrided.[66] Thorough and effective sharp debridement, i.e., to expose healthy, viable tissue is best undertaken by a trained healthcare professional as the procedure carries a high level of clinical risk.[71] There are existing frameworks for knowledge- and competency-based practice guidelines for nurses wishing to undertake

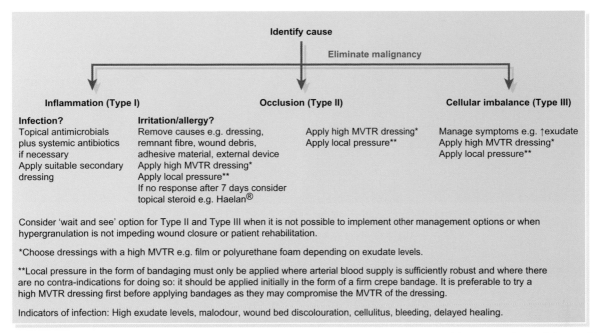

Identify cause

Eliminate malignancy

Inflammation (Type I)   **Occlusion (Type II)**   **Cellular imbalance (Type III)**

Infection?
Topical antimicrobials
plus systemic antibiotics
if necessary
Apply suitable secondary
dressing

Irritation/allergy?
Remove causes e.g. dressing,
remnant fibre, wound debris,
adhesive material, external device
Apply high MVTR dressing*
Apply local pressure**
If no response after 7 days consider
topical steroid e.g. Haelan®

Apply high MVTR dressing*
Apply local pressure**

Manage symptoms e.g. ↑exudate
Apply high MVTR dressing*
Apply local pressure**

Consider 'wait and see' option for Type II and Type III when it is not possible to implement other management options or when hypergranulation is not impeding wound closure or patient rehabilitation.

*Choose dressings with a high MVTR e.g. film or polyurethane foam depending on exudate levels.

**Local pressure in the form of bandaging must only be applied where arterial blood supply is sufficiently robust and where there are no contra-indications for doing so: it should be applied initially in the form of a firm crepe bandage. It is preferable to try a high MVTR dressing first before applying bandages as they may compromise the MVTR of the dressing.

Indicators of infection: High exudate levels, malodour, wound bed discolouration, cellulitus, bleeding, delayed healing.

Fig. 3.10 **Pathways for hypergranulation management.** MVTR, Moisture vapour transmission rate. (From Vuolo J. Hypergranulation: exploring possible management options. *Br J Nurs.* 2010;19(Tissue Viability Supplement):S4,S6-8, with permission.)

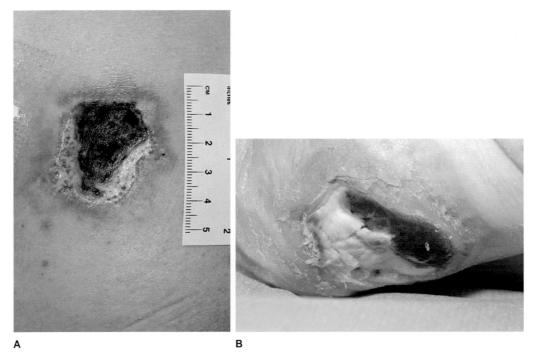

A   B

Fig. 3.11 (A) Necrotic and (B) sloughy wound.

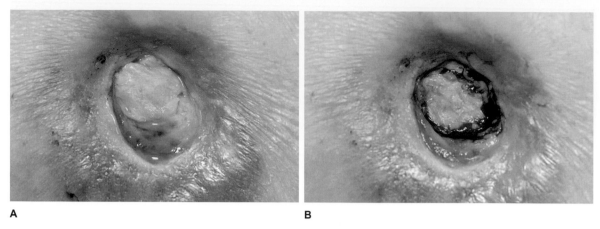

A   **B**

Fig. 3.12 Sharp debridement, (A) before and (B) after.

sharp debridement.[72] Regrettably, for some patients access to a healthcare professional competent to perform debridement is not possible, especially when patients are being cared for in the community, and a conservative approach is required. Nurses should refer to their professional code of conduct for guiding principles related to competency.

Autolytic Debridement

This is probably the most common method used in clinical practice. Autolysis refers to the process by which the body's own enzymes break down and remove dead, sloughy tissue.[73] Hydrogels and hydrocolloids effectively rehydrate devitalized tissue. In the presence of sufficient moisture, autolysis of devitalized tissue takes place. With prolonged use of moist dressings, the autolytic processes will facilitate separation of viable from non-viable tissue. This process occurs by the action of phagocytic cells and proteolytic enzymes that soften and liquefy necrotic tissue so that it can be digested by macrophages.[73] For autolysis to proceed a moist, vascular wound environment is required.[74]

Biosurgical (Maggot) Debridement

There is an increasing interest in the use of maggots for wound debridement. Therapeutic maggot therapy involves the use of the *Lucilia sericata* (greenbottle fly).[75] The mechanism by which maggots are thought to work is via the proteolytic enzymes that they secrete, which breaks down dead tissue.[75] Now available in a

'bagged form', the maggots are applied for 3–5 days where they undertake a selective and rapid form of debridement (Fig. 3.13). They are not suitable for hard, necrotic eschar or where high levels of exudate are present.[75] It is important to discuss this treatment with the patient to prepare them adequately, although previous concerns about the use of loose maggots have largely been overcome by the newer presentation within a sealed bag. Despite relatively wide acceptance by both healthcare professionals and patients, the evidence to support the superiority of maggots over other forms of debridement is lacking.[75]

There is now increasing interest in the antimicrobial capacity of secretions from maggots, specifically their action against Gram-positive bacteria.[76]

Mechanical Debridement

Methods of mechanical debridement for superficial wounds with loose slough and debris include the use of monofilament debridement pads.[77] This method is convenient, easy to use and is well tolerated by patients. Other forms of mechanical debridement include the use of a high-pressure jet of saline to remove the dead tissue, referred to as 'hydrosurgery'. This method requires training as it is very specialized.[69] Whilst not a common form of debridement, low-frequency ultrasound can be used as a safe form of debridement. However the equipment is expensive and requires very specific infection control measures. Currently the evidence to support its routine use is limited.[69] A traditional but outdated method of

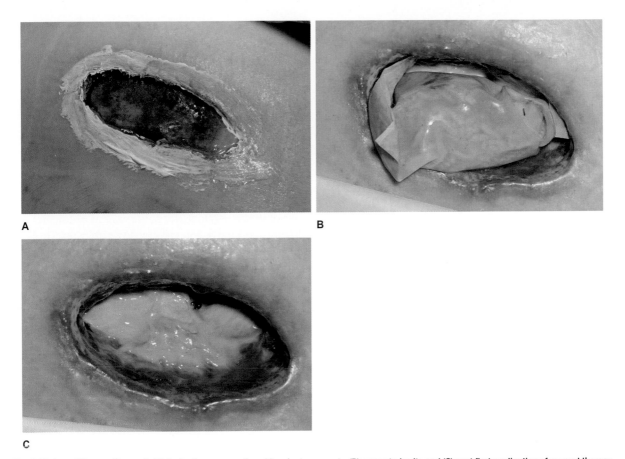

Fig. 3.13 Larval therapy (bagged). (A) Protecting surrounding skin prior to maggots, (B) maggots *in situ*, and (C) post first application of maggot therapy.

debridement is the use of wet-to-dry gauze. Essentially it involves applying a wet dressing to a wound and leaving it to dry out. As it dries it adheres to the wound bed facilitating removal of dead tissue. However the process is non-selective and carries the risk of damaging healing tissue.[68] It is also extremely painful and should be avoided.[68]

Chemical Debridement

Enzymatic agents can be applied topically to wound beds containing devitalized tissue. Such enzymatic agents are sourced from fish, fruit, animals and bacteria.[74] They can be categorized by the tissue type they target, namely proteolytic, fibronolytic or collagenase.[66] It is recommended that the skin surrounding the wound is protected by using a barrier ointment because some enzymes can damage healthy

BOX 3.3 WHEN TO SEEK SPECIALIST ADVICE

- Dry, necrotic tissue or gangrene.
- Presence of ischaemia in the lower limb.
- Terminally ill patients.
- Wounds to the face, hands, feet and genitalia.
- Wounds in close proximity to blood vessels, nerves and tendons.

skin. A secondary dressing is required with the use of enzymatic agents, with most currently used dressings being suitable. However, silver-impregnated, iodine- and zinc-based dressings should be avoided.[78] Currently the use of enzymatic dressings outside of North America is limited due to lack of availability.[73]

Specialist advice should be sought in the circumstances listed in Box 3.3.[68]

Managing Wound Infection/Bioburden

Management of wound infection presents nurses with difficult challenges. In health, host defences often resist all but the most pathogenic organisms but in ill health this ability is diminished.[55] Development of a wound infection can cause systemic problems, delay healing and result in prolonged hospital stays, particularly in relation to surgical site infections (SSIs).[79]

SURGICAL SITE INFECTION

SSI has been defined as infection that occurs at the site of surgery within 30 days of surgery, or within 1 year if an implant has been inserted.[80] SSI can be categorized into superficial, which only involves the skin and subcutaneous tissue of the incision, and deep, which involves the deep soft tissues.[81]

Sutured wounds that develop a localized infection often discharge spontaneously, so draining the infection. It may be necessary to remove one or two sutures to facilitate complete drainage. A specimen of pus can be sent for culture and sensitivity if antibiotic therapy is being considered. Once the pus has been drained, a packing material such as an alginate rope can be inserted into the wound to maintain drainage and allow the wound to heal from its depths.

When drainage of the abscess is not complete, surgical incision may be required, especially if the abscess is deep-seated; again, a dressing is used to ensure healing from the base of the wound.

RECOGNIZING INFECTION IN WOUNDS HEALING BY SECONDARY INTENTION

Local Infection

Ideally signs of an impending infection should be identified at an early stage to facilitate prompt management. The Wound Infection Institute has recently revised information related to the phases of infection[82] (Fig. 3.14), which includes a revised description for subtle (covert) and classic (overt) signs of local infection. It is at the point of identification of local infection that intervention is required to reduce the risk of spreading infection.

Spreading Infection

Spreading infection is usually seen as spreading erythema (cellulitis) (Fig. 3.15) but is also accompanied by extending induration, crepitus (cracking or popping) on palpation and lymphangitis.[82] Patients may also report symptoms such as a general malaise, lethargy and loss of appetite.

Prompt treatment with systemic and topical antimicrobials is required to avoid the sequelae of a systemic inflammatory response (SIR), i.e., sepsis, leading to death.[82]

DEVICES AND ADVANCED INTERVENTIONS FOR MANAGEMENT OF WOUNDS

Whilst uncomplicated wounds generally heal with the use of dressings alone, for some wound aetiologies the use of adjunctive interventions/therapies are needed as part of the standard management plan (Table 3.3). Piaggesi et al.[1] defines these advanced wound therapies as:

… therapies based on novel principles and technologies, or in reference to a novel application of consolidated principles and technologies, including either a singular mechanism of action or a strategy with different levels of action …

These authors group these advanced therapies into four main categories:
- materials (advanced wound dressings)
- cell and tissue engineering
- physical and biophysical
- sensors and IT-related measures.

In terms of materials, commonly available dressings have already been addressed. However, there are also more advanced materials such as acellular matrices, which have been designed to replace or promote extracellular matrix formation. These can be naturally derived from animal or human tissue and can be used on a range of different wounds such as burn injuries, diabetic foot ulcers and venous leg ulcers.

Cell and tissue engineering (regenerative medicine) is also an emerging area of wound management where a number of cell types are being explored (Table 3.4).

Tissue-based therapies contain living cells, either from the patient themselves (autologous) or from other humans (allogenic). These can contain epidermis, dermis or both (dermo-epidermal) and may be permanent or temporary. None of the tissue-based therapies are suitable for use on infected wounds. Therefore this would need treating before considering their use.[1]

'Physical' therapies to enhance wound healing include some of the modalities already discussed, i.e., mechanical debridement interventions, compression therapy and negative-pressure wound therapy (NPWT). Additionally, there is increasing interest

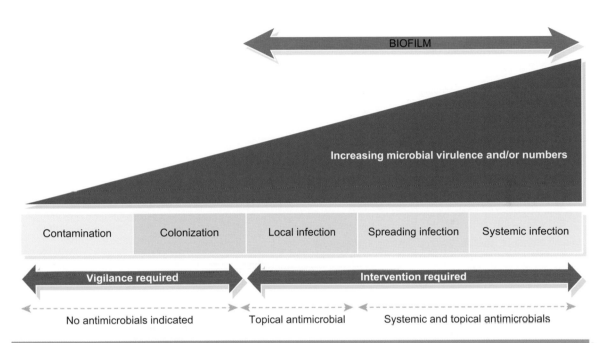

Contamination[26]	Colonization[26]	Local infection		Spreading infection[22,23]	Systemic infection[22,23]
All wounds may acquire micro-organisms. If suitable nutritive and physical conditions are not available for each microbial species, or they are not able to successfully evade host defences, they will not multiply or persist; their presence is therefore only transient and wound healing is not delayed	Microbial species successfully grow and divide, but do not cause damage to the host or initiate wound infection	Covert (subtle) signs of local infection:[2,27-36] ■ Hypergranulation (excessive 'vascular' tissue) ■ Bleeding, friable granulation ■ Epithelial bridging and pocketing in granulation tissue ■ Wound breakdown and enlargement ■ Delayed wound healing beyond expectations ■ New or increasing pain ■ Increasing malodour	Overt (classic) signs of local infection:[2,27,28,35,36] ■ Erythema ■ Local warmth ■ Swelling ■ Purulent discharge ■ Delayed wound healing beyond expectations ■ New or increasing pain ■ Increasing malodour	■ Extending in duration +/– erythema ■ Lymphangitis ■ Crepitus ■ Wound breakdown/ dehiscence with or without satellite lesions ■ Malaise/ lethargy or non specific general deterioration ■ Loss of appetite ■ Inflammation, swelling of lymph glands	■ Severe sepsis ■ Septic shock ■ Organ failure ■ Death

Table 1: Signs and symptoms associated with stages of the wound infection continuum

A

Continued

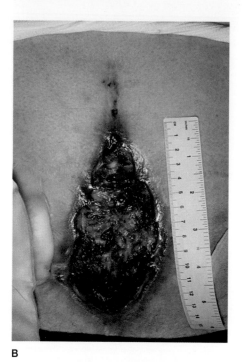

B

Fig. 3.14 **(A)** Phases of infection. **(B)** Local infection in a dehisced wound abdominal wound. (A, From the International Wound Infection Institute, with permission.)

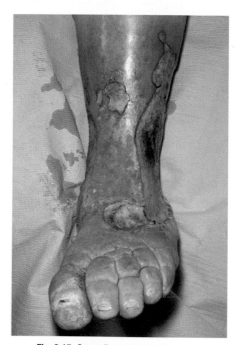

Fig. 3.15 Spreading erythema/cellulitis.

TABLE 3.3	Adjunctive Interventions/ Therapies for the Management of Wounds
Aetiology	**Best Practice Management**
Venous leg ulcer	Compression therapy – including the use of bandages, hosiery, wraps/ garments
Diabetic foot ulcers	Footwear and off-loading interventions – including casts and prefabricated devices (non-removable/ removable), therapeutic footwear[a]
Pressure ulcers/ pressure injuries	Pressure redistributing equipment – including mattresses and cushions[b]
Wound healing by primary and secondary intention	Negative-pressure wound therapy – for closed, incisional and open wound management and can be used with instillation to manage infection

[a]IWGDF *Guideline on offloading foot ulcers in persons with diabetes*, 2019. Available at: https://iwgdfguidelines.org/offloading-guideline/

[b]National Pressure Ulcer Advisory Panel, European Pressure Ulcer Advisory Panel and Pan Pacific Pressure Injury Alliance. *Prevention and Treatment of Pressure Ulcers: Quick Reference Guide*. Perth, Australia: Cambridge Media. 2014. Available at: http://www.epuap.org/pu-guidelines/

and use of oxygen therapy (via hyperbaric or topical means) and electrical stimulation to augment standard care. Newer technologies under current investigation include use of extracorporeal shock wave therapy, electromagnetic fields, photo-biomodulation (light therapy) and nanotechnology.[1] Proponents of these emerging technologies suggest they show promise, but currently the initial costs preclude adoption into clinical practice. However there is an economic argument for advanced interventions when the direct and indirect costs of standard treatments are taken into account.

TABLE 3.4   Stem Cells and Other Therapeutically Active Cells

Cell Type	Advantages	Disadvantages
Bone marrow stem cells	Able to differentiate in any cell line	Difficult to retrieve and only obtainable in small quantities
Keratinocytes and fibro-blasts	Obtainable from skin biopsies	Requires a relatively long culture time, tissue is fragile, suitable for small areas only
Adipose-derived stem cells	Easy to obtain, can differentiate in any cell line, good regenerative and volumetric capacity	Contraindicated in cancer diseases
Platelets	Contains essential growth factors, can be used as medium to support other cell therapies	Minimal – but does require a blood sample to be obtained (20 cc)
Leucocytes	Contains essential growth factors, antibacterial, capable of modifying the immune response, co-ordinates wound healing	Minimal – but does require a blood sample to be obtained (20 cc)
Monocytes	Shown to enhance neovascularization, easy to obtain, differentiation has been shown *in vitro*	No differentiation in epithelial cells *in vivo*
Epithelial stem cell (hair follicle)	Easy to obtain	Limited evidence to demonstrate effect

Adapted from Piaggesi A, Läuchli S, Biedermann BF, et al. Advanced therapies in wound management: cell and tissue based therapies, physical and bio-physical therapies smart and IT based technologies. *J Wound Care*. 2018;27(6):S1–S137.

Summary

Although wound interventions are becoming more and more sophisticated, the basis of managing any wound successfully is as outlined in this chapter.

Before moving on to the case studies in the rest of the book, ensure that you have understood the following basic principles:

- The development of dressing materials
  - Moist wound healing
  - Range of modern dressings, devices and adjunctive therapies
- Management of wounds healing by primary and secondary intention
  - Signs of local (covert and overt) and spreading infection
  - Wound debridement
  - Moisture balance
- Prevention of infection
  - Aseptic Non-Touch Technique (ANTT)
  - Hand washing
- Wound cleansing
  - Indications for cleansing
  - Methods of cleansing

REFERENCES

1. Piaggesi A, Läuchli S, Bassetto F, et al. Advanced therapies in wound management: cell and tissue based therapies, physical and bio-physical therapies smart and IT based technologies. *J Wound Care*. 2018;27(6):S1–S137.
2. Majino G. *The Healing Hand: Man and Wound in the Ancient World*. Cambridge, MA: Harvard University Press; 1975.
3. Broughton G, Janis JE, Attinger CE. The basic science of wound healing plast. *Reconstr Surg*. 2006;117(7S):12S–34S.
4. Leaper DJ. History of Wound Healing. In: Leaper DJ, Harding KG, eds. *Wounds Biology and Management*. Oxford: Oxford University Press; 1998:5–9.
5. Dealey C. Wound management products. In: Dealey C, ed. *The Care of Wounds: A Guide for Nurses*. 4th ed. Oxford: Wiley Blackwell; 2012:93–110.
6. Freiberg JA. The mythos of laudable pus along with an explanation for its origin. *J Community Hosp Intern Med Perspect*. 2017;7(3):196–198.
7. Naylor IL. Ulcer care in the Middle Ages. *J Wound Care*. 1999;8(4):208–212.
8. Crumplin M. Medical aspects of the Waterloo campaign of 1815. *RCS Bull*. 2016;98(2):70–73.
9. Smith KA. Louis Pasteur, the Father of Immunology? *Front Immunol*. 2012;3:68.
10. Pitt D, Aubin JM. Joseph Lister: father of modern surgery. *Can J Surg*. 2012;55(5):E8–E9.
11. Lister J. On the antiseptic principle in the practice of surgery. *Br Med J*. 1867;2(351):246–248.
12. Tröhler U. Statistics and the British controversy about the effects of Joseph Lister's system of antisepsis for surgery, 1867–1890. *J R Soc Med*. 2015;108(7):280–287.

13. Leaper DJ. *Eusol. BMJ.* 1992;304(11):930–931.
14. Cornwell P, Arnold-Long M, Barss SB, Varnado MF. The use of dakin's solution in chronic wounds: a clinical perspective case series. *J Wound Ostomy Continence Nurs.* 2010;37(1):94–104.
15. Rhodes P. *An Outline History of Medicine.* London: Butterworths; 1986.
16. Lobanovska M, Pilla G. Drug development penicillin's discovery and antibiotic resistance: lessons for the future? *Yale J Biol Med.* 2017;90(1):135–145.
17. Turk JL. Leonard Colebrook: the chemotherapy and control of streptococcal infections. *J Royal Soc Med.* 1994;87:727–728.
18. Lowbury EJL. Leonard Colebrook (1883-1967). *J Hosp Infect.* 1983;4:330.
19. Dhivya S, Padma VV, Santhini E. *Wound dressings – a review Biomedicine (Taipei).* 2015;5(4):22.
20. Romanovsky AA. Paracelsus on wound treatment. *Lancet.* 1999;354:1910.
21. Drucker CB. Ambroise paré and the birth of the gentle art of surgery. *Yale J Biol Med.* 2008;81(4):199–202.
22. Markatos K, Tzivra A, Tsoutsos S, Tsourouflis G, Karamanou M, Androutsos G. Ambroise Paré (1510-1590) and his innovative work on the treatment of war injuries. *Surgi Innov.* 2018;25(2):183–186.
23. Kapadia HM. Sampson Gamgee: a great Birmingham surgeon. *J Royal Soc Med.* 2002;95:96–100.
24. Rajendran S. *Advanced Textiles for Wound Care.* 2nd ed. Duxford Woodhead Publishing, Elsevier; 2019.
25. Winter GD. Formation of the scab and rate of epithelialization of superficial wounds in the skin of the young domestic pig. *Nature.* 1962;193:293–294.
26. Dyson M, Young S, Pendle C. Comparison of the effects of moist and dry conditions on dermal repair. *J Invest Dermatol.* 1988;91(5):435–439.
27. Hinman C, Maibach H. Effects of air exposure and occlusion on experimental human skin wounds. *Nature.* 1963;2000:377–378.
28. Turner TD. Semiocclusive and occlusive dressings. In: Ryan TJ, ed. *An Environment for Healing: the Role of Occlusion. Royal Society of Medicine Congress and Symposium Series 8.* London: Royal Society of Medicine Press; 1985.
29. Thomas S. *Functions of a wound dressing.* In: *Wound Management and Dressings.* London: The Pharmaceutical Press; 1990.
30. Bale S, Morison M. Wound dressings. In: Morison M, Moffatt C, Bridel-Nixon J, Bale S, eds. *A Colour Guide to the Nursing Management of Chronic Wounds.* London: Mosby; 1997.
31. Thomas S, Leigh I. Wound dressings. I: Leaper DJ, Harding KG, eds. *Wounds Biology and Management.* Oxford: Oxford University Press; 1998:166–183.
32. Baranoski S, Ayello EA. Wound dressings: an evolving art and science. *Adv Skin Wound Care.* 2012;25(2):87–92.
33. Schultz GS, Sibbald RG, Falanga V, et al. Wound bed preparation: a systematic approach to wound management. *Wound Rep Reg.* 2003;11:1–28.
34. Leaper DJ, Schultz G, Carville K, Fletcher J, Swanson T, Drake R. Extending the TIME concept: what have we learned in the past 10 years? *Int Wound J.* 2014;9(Suppl. 2):1–19.
35. Harries RI., Bosanquet DC, Harding KG. Wound bed preparation: TIME for an update. *Int Wound J.* 2016;13(Suppl. S3):8–14.
36. Holloway S, Harding K, Stechmiller J, Schultz G. Acute and chronic wound healing. In: Baranoski S, Ayello EA, eds. *Wound Care Essentials.* 4th ed. Philadelphia: Wolters Kluwer; 2016.
37. Atkin L, Bućko Z, Conde Montero E, et al. Implementing TIMERS: the race against hard-to-heal wounds. *J Wound Care.* 2019;1(Sup3a, 23):S1–S50.
38. Holloway S, Harding KG. Wounds. In: Whittlesea C, Hodson K, eds. *Clinical Pharmacy and Therapeutics.* 6th ed. China: Elsevier; 2019:1017–1034.
39. Stryja J, Sandy-Hodgetts K, Collier M, et al. Surgical site infection: preventing and managing surgical site infection across health care sectors. *J Wound Care.* 2020;29:2(suppl 2b):S1–S69.
40. National Institute of Health and Clinical Excellence. *Surgical Site Infection.* London: National Institute of Health and Clinical Excellence; 2013. Available at: https://www.nice.org.uk/guidance/qs49/resources/surgical-site-infection-pdf-2098675107781.
41. Vowden K, Vowden P. Wound dressings: principles and practice. *Surg.* 2017;35(9):489–494.
42. Chrintz H, Vibits H, Cordtz TO, Harreby JS, Waaddegaard P, Larsen SO. Need for surgical wound dressing. *Br J Surg.* 1989;76:204–205.
43. Lusuku C, Ramamoorthy R, Davidson BR, Gurusamy KS. Early versus delayed dressing removal after primary closure of clean and clean-contaminated surgical wounds. *Cochrane Database Syst Rev.* 2015;9:CD010259.
44. Milne J, Vowden P, Fumarola S, Leaper D. *Postoperative incision management made easy;* 2012. Wounds UK suppl. 8(4), Available at: www.wounds-uk.com/made-easy.
45. National Institute for Health and Care Excellence (NICE). *Infection prevention and control.* London: NICE; 2014. Available at: https://www.nice.org.uk/guidance/qs61.
46. European Centre for Disease Prevention and Control (ECDC). *Organisation of infection prevention and control in healthcare settings.* Solna, Sweden: ECDC; 2015. Available at: https://ecdc.europa.eu/en/publications-data/directory-guidance-prevention-and-control/measures-in-hospitals.
47. World Health Organization (WHO). *Guidelines on core components of infection prevention and control programmes at the national and acute health care facility level.* Geneva: WHO; 2016. Available at: https://www.who.int/gpsc/ipc-components/en/.
48. Boyce J-M, Pittet D. Guidelines for hand hygiene in healthcare settings: recommendations of the healthcare infection control practices advisory committee and the HICPAC/SHEA/APIC/IDSA hand hygiene task force. Centre for Disease Control. *Morb Mortal Wkly Rep.* 2002;17(51):1–45.
49. Sax H, Allegranzi B, Uçkay I, Larson E, Boyce J, Pittet D. 'My five moments for hand hygiene': a user-centred design approach to understand, train, monitor and report hand hygiene. *J Hosp Infect.* 2007;67(1):9–21.
50. Rowley S. Aseptic non touch technique nursing times. *Infection Control Supplement.* 2001;97(7):V1–V111.
51. Rowley S, Clare S. ANTT: a standard approach to aseptic technique. *Nurs Times.* 2011;107(36):12–14.
52. Lloyd-Jones M. Wound cleansing: is it necessary, or just a ritual? *Nurs Residential Care.* 2012;14(8):396–399.
53. Stotts NA. Wound infection: diagnosis and management. In: Bryant RA, Nix D, eds. *Acute and Chronic Wounds: Nursing Management.* 5th ed. St. Louis, MO: Elsevier; 2016:283–294.
54. Cutting KF, White RJ. Maceration of the skin and wound bed 1: its nature and causes. *J Wound Care.* 2002;11(7):275–278.
55. Stotts NA. Bioburden infection. In: Baranoski S, Ayello EA, eds. *Wound Care Essentials.* 4th ed. Philadelphia: Wolters Kluwers; 2016:121–148.

56. Towler J. Cleansing traumatic wounds with swabs, water or saline. *J Wound Care.* 2001;10(6):231–234.

57. Hayek S, El Khatib A, Atiyeh B. Burn wound cleansing - a myth or a scientific practice. *Ann Burns Fire Disasters.* 2010;23(1):19–24.

58. Bryant RA, Nix D. Principles of wound healing and topical management. In: Bryant RA, Nix D, eds. *Acute and Chronic Wounds: Nursing Management.* 5th ed. St. Louis, MO: Elsevier; 306–324.

59. Hellewell TB, Major DA, Rodeheaver PF, Rodeheaver GT. Cytotoxicity evaluation of antimicrobial and non-antimicrobial wound cleansers. *Wounds.* 9(1):15–20.

60. Fernandez R, Griffiths R. Water for wound cleansing. *Cochrane Database Syst Rev.* 2012;2:CD003861.

61. Roberts CD, Leaper DJ, Assadian O. The role of topical antiseptic agents within antimicrobial stewardship strategies for prevention and treatment of surgical site and chronic open wound infection. *Adv Wound Care.* 2017;6(2):63–71.

62. Vermeulen H, Ubbink DT, Goossens A, de Vos R, Legemate DA, Westerbos SJ. Dressings and topical agents to help surgical wounds heal by secondary intention. *Br J Surg.* 2005;92:665–672.

63. Heinrichs EL, Llewellyn M, Harding K. Assessment of a patient with a wound. In: Gray D, Cooper P, eds. *Wound Healing: A Systematic Approach to Advanced Wound Healing and Management.* 2005:1–27.

64. Falanga V, Brem H, Ennis WJ, Wolcott R, Gould LJ, Ayello EA. Maintenance debridement in the treatment of difficult-to-heal chronic wounds. Recommendations of an expert panel. *Ostomy Wound Manage.* 2008;(Suppl):2e13.

65. Caley MP, Martins VLC, O'Toole EA. Metalloproteinases and wound healing. *Adv Wound Care.* 2015;4(4):225–234.

66. Ayello EA, Sibbald RG, Baranoski S. Wound debridement. In: Ayello EA, Baranoski S, eds. *Wound Care Essentials.* Philadelphia: Wolters Kluwer; 2016:149–170.

67. Vuolo J. Hypergranulation: exploring possible management options. *Br J Nurs.* 2010;19(6):S4–S8. Tissue Viability Supplement.

68. Lloyd-Jones M. Wound debridement, part 2. *Br J Healthcare Assistants.* 2018;12(3):115–117.

69. Mahoney J, Ward J. Surgical debridement. In: Teot L, Banwell PE, Ziegler UE, eds. *Surgery in Wounds.* Berlin: Springer-Verlag; 2004:67–71.

70. Schwartz JA, Goss SG, Facchin F, Avdagic E, Lantis JC. Surgical debridement alone does not adequately reduce planktonic bioburden in chronic lower extremity wounds. *J Wound Care.* 2014;23(9). S4, S6, S8 passim.

71. Bentley J, Bishai P, Foster A, Preece J. Clinical competence in sharp debridement: an innovative course. *Wound Care.* 2005:S6–S13.

72. Fairbairn K, Grier J, Hunter C, Preece J. A sharp debridement procedure devised by specialist nurses. *J Wound Care.* 2002;11(10):371–375.

73. Vowden P. Autolytic debridement. In: Teot L, Banwell PE, Ziegler UE, eds. *Surgery in Wounds.* Berlin: Springer-Verlag; 2004:77–80.

74. Ramundo JM. Wound debridement. In: Bryant RA, Nix DP, eds. *Acute and Chronic Wounds.* 5th ed. St. Louis, MO: Elsevier; 2016:295–305.

75. Shi E, Shofler D. Maggot debridement therapy: a systematic review. *Br J Community Nurs.* 2014:S6–13. Suppl Wound Care.

76. Jaklic D, Lapanje A, Zupancic K, Smrke D, Gunde-Cimerman N. Selective antimicrobial activity of maggots against pathogenic bacteria Domen. *J Med Microbiol.* 2008;57:617–662.

77. National Institute for Health and Care Excellence (NICE). *The Debrisoft monofilament debridement pad for use in acute or chronic wounds. MTG17.* London: NICE; 2014. Available at: https://www.nice.org.uk/guidance/mtg17.

78. Shi L, Ermis R, Kiedaisch B, Carson D. The effect of various wound dressings on the activity of debriding enzymes. *Adv Skin Wound Care.* 2010;23(10):456–462.

79. Badia JM, Casey AL, Petrosillo N, Hudson PM, Mitchell SA, Crosby C. Impact of surgical site infection on healthcare costs and patient outcomes: a systematic review in six European countries. *J Hosp Infect.* 2017;96(1):1–15.

80. National Institute for Health and Care Excellence (NICE). *Surgical Site Infection.* London: NICE; 2008. Available at: https://www.nice.org.uk/guidance/cg74/evidence/full-guideline 242005933.

81. Berríos-Torres SI, Umscheid CA, Bratzler DW, et al. Centers for Disease Control and Prevention Guideline for the Prevention of Surgical Site Infection. *JAMA Surg.* 2017;152(8):784–791.

82. Ousey K, Haesler E. Evolution of the wound infection Continuum. *Wounds International.* 2018;9(4):6–10. Available at: www.woundsinternational.com.

FURTHER READING

Baranoski S, Ayello AE. *Wound Care Essentials: Practice Principles.* Philadelphia: Wolters Kluwer; 2016.

Bryant RA, Nix DP. *Acute and Chronic Wounds: Current Management Concepts.* St. Louis, MO: Elsevier; 2016.

Edwards-Jones V. *Essential Microbiology for Wound Care.* Oxford: Oxford University Press; 2016.

Flanagan M. *Wound Healing and Skin Integrity.* Chichester: Wiley-Blackwell; 2013.

MCQS

1 *Which of the following statements about the management of an uncomplicated wound healing by primary intention is false?*

a. Sterile saline should be used for cleansing postoperative wounds
b. Showering is permissible 48 hours after surgery
c. Daily dressing changes are required
d. Topical antimicrobial agents should not be used

2 *Appropriate methods of debridement include:*
a. Hydrogels and hydrocolloids to promote autolysis
b. Sharp debridement
c. Maggots
d. Wet-to-dry gauze

3 *Subtle signs of local infection include:*
a. Spreading cellulitis
b. Wound dehiscence/breakdown
c. Increasing pain
d. Bleeding, friable tissue

Chapter 4

Wound Care in the Baby and Young Child

Anna-Barbara Schlüer

Highlights

- Severe and long lasting wounds are mostly limited to chronic conditions or after severe burns in paediatric patients
- It is a clinical challenge to find dressings that are appropriate both to the goal that has to be achieved in wound healing and to specific paediatric needs
- In addition, the choice of a dressing in children should be regularly evaluated
- Paediatric patients are not small adults, and this is also true for wound care

Key Issues

This is the first of the life-cycle chapters and deals with the neonate, baby and young child. As you read through this chapter concentrate on the following:
- The choice of dressings that will alleviate pain and minimize trauma and scarring
- The size and type of dressing suitable for babies and small children
- The ways in which nurses can interact with parents and children to decrease emotional trauma
- The importance of documentation of the wound, however small

Introduction

The United Nations Convention on the Rights of the Child defines a child as 'a human being below the age of 18 years'.[1] Within this time period we distinguish between neonate, infant, toddler, preschool child, school child and adolescent[2]:
- Neonate: a child from birth up until his/her first 30 days of life; this includes:

- preterm neonate: born before 38 weeks of gestational age
- term-born neonate: born after 37 weeks of gestational age
- newborn: a neonate within his/her first hours of life
- Infant: a child from the age of 4 weeks up to his/her first birthday
- Toddler: a child from the age of 1 year up to his/her third birthday
- Preschool child: a child between 3 and 5 years of age
- School child: a child between 6 and 12 years of age
- Adolescent: covers the time from 12 years up to the 18th birthday.

It should be kept in mind that paediatric patients differ widely in health conditions compared to adults. The overall health status of children is generally better and multi-morbidity is limited to a small percentage of patients, such as very low-term neonates (born before 32 weeks of gestation age), newborns with congenital abnormalities, chromosomopathies, perinatal distress syndrome or children with chronic conditions. Survival rates of both critically and chronically ill neonates, infants and children have improved dramatically in recent years, introducing new challenges for medical and nursing care. Furthermore, new devices, extracorporeal membrane oxygenation (ECMO), long-lasting surgical procedures and advanced therapies in critical and emergency care require much more attention in order to prevent pressure-related ulcers.[3]

In infants the neonatal period covers the first 4 weeks of life. When considering the whole life-cycle, the neonatal period is the most hazardous, with high mortality. The neonatal mortality rate is defined as the number of liveborn infants who die before the age of 28 days per 1000 births in the same year. Although neonatal mortality in England and Wales remained in 2014 the same as in 2013, 6.7 deaths per thousand total births, 2.7 deaths per thousand live births, 1.2 deaths per thousand live births and respectively. Between 1984 and 2014, the neonatal mortality rates fell by 52%.[4] For neonates the first day of life is critical – more neonates die on the first day than during the period from 12 months to 25 years.

It follows that caring for neonates and infants with wounds presents nurses with many difficult problems. The most obvious are the smallness and vulnerability of the neonate. In babies born prematurely this is even more pronounced.

The main causes of death in children include accidents, congenital abnormalities and cancers.[5] The young child with a wound and wound problems also has special requirements.

The Skin in Paediatrics: From Fetus to Newborn

When it comes to wound care in paediatric patients we need to be familiar with paediatric skin morphology and physiology. The most important function of the skin is to protect against water loss, absorption of noxious substances, invasion of microorganisms and physical trauma.[6] The skin of children is morphologically and functionally different from adult skin.[6–8] Within the first days of life neonates undergo various adaptation processes needed to accommodate the transition from the wet intrauterine environment to the dry outside environment.[6] During the first months and years the skin continues to develop and evolve its structure and function.

There are unique physiological needs of children with regard to skin. Physiologically, fluid and electrolyte disturbances occur more frequently and develop more rapidly in infants and young children than in older children and adults. The higher proportion of water content and greater relative surface area of young bodies increases the risk of dehydration under the metabolic demands associated with fever. Skin cells that are not well perfused may be hypoxic and are at risk of breaking down even with minimal trauma. The skin barrier evolves its structure after about 14 life days in the neonate.

It is known that any skin breakdown, especially in critically ill neonates and infants, increases the risk of septicaemia, as well as related severe complications and higher mortality.[9] Therefore it is of great importance to avoid any damage to the fragile skin of paediatric patients.

This is a challenging area of nursing and one in which the creativity and skills of the nurse can be pivotal in producing the best possible outcome for the child. The principles of caring for sick children must be considered in conjunction with all the principles of managing patients with wounds as previously discussed.[10]

In this chapter the principles of managing sick children are dealt with only in relation to issues specific to wound management. Further reading on the management of sick children can be found in paediatric nursing textbooks (see Further Reading).

Nursing Infants

When serious illness occurs, the family is often thrown into physical and emotional crisis. With support, many stable families are able to cope, although less stable ones may experience great difficulties.[11] The paediatric ward staff are highly trained in understanding the needs of, and in caring for, the whole family when an infant is admitted to hospital. On admission the immediate goals of the staff include:

- gaining the parents' cooperation and trust
- alleviating anxiety or restoring it to an acceptable level
- preserving the relationships between the parents and infant.[10]

Nurses achieve these goals by:

- explaining all the medical and nursing procedures and enlisting the help and support of parents to promote a feeling of partnership between staff and parents
- encouraging parents to stay with their baby for as long as possible or to visit at any time of the day or night (it is usual for beds or chairs to be provided for parents at the infant's bedside, so that they need not be separated)
- helping the parents to understand that regression often occurs. Boredom can also be a problem for infants. This can be helped by placing interesting toys near the child, by talking and interacting with the child whenever they are close and by

allowing siblings and other older children to play with or around the child.

However, hospitalization is being reduced as much as possible and increasing numbers of children are being cared for at home as this is considered to be the best environment.[12] Whatever the physical environment a baby or child is nursed in, it is important that they are carefully assessed.[13] One of the main principles of nursing sick children is to meet the needs of the child as an individual.[11] This involves:

- recognizing each child as a unique, developing individual whose best interests must be paramount
- listening to the child, attempting to understand his/her perspective, opinions and feelings, and acknowledging his/her right to privacy[14]
- considering the physical, psychological, social, cultural and spiritual needs of the child and his/her family[11]
- respecting the right of the child, according to his/her age and understanding, to appropriate information and informed participation in decisions about their care.[15]

The role of the child's family is an important factor in planning the wound care of an individual child.[16] As healthcare is shared with the family, the parents can become actively involved in delivering wound care to their child. Although it is important to recognize that not all parents will want to become actively involved, the majority can feel happy and comfortable about delivering basic wound care. In this situation the nurse provides the education and support that enables parents to learn the necessary skills.

Pain

Assessment of a child's pain and the subsequent effective management of that pain can be extremely difficult.[17] In children, acute pain can result in restlessness and agitation, tachycardia, hypertension, pupil dilation, crying and being difficult to comfort.

Historical attitudes to children's experiences of pain are interesting. Although much research had been undertaken on pain in the adult, it was not until the 1970s that pain was considered to be an important issue in paediatrics.[11]

Children may have difficulties in expressing and communicating to others that they are in pain and also in describing what sort of pain they have.[18] With careful observation nurses and parents can help assess a child's pain in three ways:

- by listening carefully to the child; young children may use a variety of different phrases to express that they are in pain, whereas older children can be quite specific
- by observing changes in the child's behaviour (the parent may report such changes)
- the child may show physiological signs of pain such as increased pulse rate, raised blood pressure and respiratory rate.

Visual scales have been developed to help children express their level of pain and assess the effectiveness of pharmacological and psychological methods of relieving pain.[11,17]

Wound management, including dressing changes, need not be associated with pain or discomfort. The nurse's skill in assessing the child with a wound should ensure that the most appropriate wound treatment and dressing are chosen to minimize trauma at dressing changes.[16]

Dressings Suitable for Children

In complex wound-care situations, dressing changes are always performed by professionals, sometimes under analgosedation. However, a ward nurse can support and encourage the parents to learn to care for the child's wound in hospital in more straightforward situations. Once the child is home the community nurse is able to continue this support. The child may wish to return to school, nursery or more normal activity before the wound is completely healed. A wide range of dressing materials is available to meet the needs of children with different wound types and problems.[19] The choice of dressing and wound care needs to be a joint decision between the child, parents and nurse. Certain dressing materials are particularly suitable for children, especially those that provide an occlusive or semiocclusive environment. As discussed in Chapter 3, these materials include semipermeable films and hydrocolloids that are self-adherent and isolate the wound from the outside environment. The child is thus able to play and bathe without the parents having to worry about the wound getting dirty or wet. For deeper, cavity wounds semipermeable films can be used to hold other dressing materials in place, for example alginates, gels and foams.

Caution is needed when applying topical agents to large areas in neonates, as absorption (for example, of calcium from alginates) may interfere with their delicate electrolyte balance. The majority of modern dressing materials are soft, conformable and comfortable and come in a wide range of sizes so that small children are well catered for.

WOUND CLEANSING AND DRESSING APPLICATION

It can be extremely difficult to perform a strict aseptic technique on a baby or small child. Small children are easily distracted and get bored and also may be frightened by a dressing pack and equipment. Even using gloves can cause some children great distress. Hands cleansed with gel can be used for wound dressing and dressing changes either by a parent or the nurse.[14] As an alternative, the use of a shower-head or bowl of water may provide a less frightening alternative to wound irrigation with a syringe and quill.[16,19] As with adults, wound cleansing and dressing changes should only be carried out when indicated. Such indications include the presence of devitalized tissue, infection or excess exudate production. Unnecessary repeated wound cleansing and dressing changes will only traumatize newly forming tissue.

RETURNING TO NORMAL ACTIVITY

Wound therapies and dressing should permit the child to have as near normal day-to-day activities as possible. To facilitate this the nurse may choose dressing materials that are not bulky or use items of clothing to hold dressings in place. In small babies, nappies can be used to hold dressings in the perineal area in place. Children may also pull or fiddle with their dressings and it may be necessary to apply a pad and bandage over the top to prevent this.

Extravasation Injury

Extravasation injuries may occur as a consequence of the difficulty of giving intravenous fluids to

---

Case Study 4.1

Extravasation Injury

Ten-day-old Samantha Marks was born at 40 weeks' gestation and was a well-developed full-term neonate. Following a normal delivery, Samantha was progressing well until 5 days after delivery she became restless and irritable, refusing to feed, and was found to be pyrexic (38°C). Microbiological examination revealed that she had a Gram-negative septicaemia that was immediately treated with a course of intravenous antibiotics, via an infusion that was sited in her left foot.

During infusion the cannula became dislodged and a large amount of antibiotic solution invaded the subcutaneous tissue of her foot. The infusion was re-sited in the right foot but the damage to the left foot resulted in an area of inflamed tissue that extended over the whole of the dorsal area (Fig. 4.1).

Initially treated with dry dressing by the paediatric nurses, within 3 days the inflamed area became necrotic and sloughy, exuding large amounts of exudate, and inflammation began to spread up Samantha's leg. The area was obviously very painful when touched and, although her general condition was now improving, the wound was causing Samantha and her parents great distress.

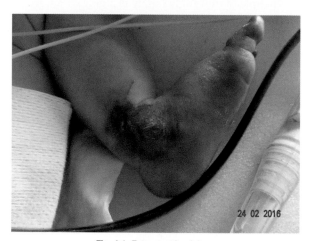

Fig. 4.1 Extravasation injury.

small children. Case Study 4.1 describes a typical problem.

AETIOLOGY

During illness some infants will require fluids to be given intravenously. Infants have a higher fluid requirement in proportion to their surface area than adults and during illness the basal metabolic rate can significantly increase. The kidneys are immature and so fluid intake must be closely monitored.[15]

In neonates an infusion may be sited in the scalp or foot, as cannulation in the cubital fossae or hands is technically difficult.[20]

Extravasation injuries are often the result of intravenous solutions leaking into the surrounding tissue. Infiltration of fluid may result in scarring or amputation with fatal consequences.[21] A higher percentage of injuries occur when infusions are sited in lower limbs and, in some situations, damage occurs to the nerves and tendons, with ensuing tissue death and necrosis.

MANAGEMENT

Should extravasation occur, the infusion must be stopped immediately, the cannula removed, the doctor alerted and the pharmacist contacted to advise on potential toxicity of the infused substance. Prevention of this type of tissue injury can be best achieved by frequent observation of the infusion site. It is therefore advisable to secure cannulae with a semipermeable film dressing rather than bandage. Nothing replaces careful observation of these sites by the nurse, as even intravenous delivery pumps are not considered reliable in detecting extravasation. Management of the resulting injury is essential, as extensive tissue death could result in further damage with disastrous consequences.

The commonest method of management is the use of a sterile foam dressing to protect the wound area and avoid further mechanical friction. In extreme cases debridement, grafting and secondary reconstruction may be necessary so it is important that nurses monitor extravasation sites by measuring and documenting the position of the injury, the amount and type of wound tissue (e.g., necrotic, sloughy or granulating) and the extent and spread of erythema.

Nursing Model for Samantha

When dealing with such a young infant, the nurse's role will depend largely on interaction with Samantha's parents. The type of nursing care given to Samantha's wound could have a profound effect on the rest of her life. The damage has already been done, but further deterioration of the wound could result in her losing the use of her foot or even the foot itself.

When choosing a model for Samantha consider the following priorities of care:

- the *trauma* to the parents of having their new baby become so ill in a short space of time
- the parents' *understanding* of the situation: do they know what has caused the injury to Samantha's foot?
- do they realize the potential problems that could arise from *mismanagement* of the wound?
- Samantha still has to *recover* fully from her septicaemia
- Samantha is experiencing *pain* when her foot is handled; this may discourage her parents from picking her up and cuddling her
- do the nurses understand the *legal* implications of this baby's care?

Look at the emphasized points: *trauma, understanding, mismanagement, recover, pain* and *legal*. All these points focus on the parents', nurse's and baby's *perceptions* of the situation. The type of environment in which the baby is nursed will greatly affect the parents' perception of this situation. An environment full of equipment and staff busying themselves with the baby may alienate the parents and they will feel they are not being told everything. Although in Samantha's case her physiological care is important, the nurse must concentrate also on the psychological and sociological parameters to help the parents deal with their baby's illness. Riehl's interaction model addresses these issues[22] and she advocates the use of the FANCAP system (fluids, aeration, nutrition, communication, activity and pain) developed by Abbey[23] to assess patient needs. This can be applied to Samantha's needs as shown in Table 4.1

Practice Points

- Some of the problems have been highlighted; can you identify any others?
- The management of the wound can be achieved with the use of a foam dressing.
- This situation should be organized by an experienced paediatric team leader, as it is essential that parents and nurses are kept informed of the implications of this type of injury.

TABLE 4.1 Use of the FANCAP Mnemonic to Plan Samantha's Care

FANCAP	Physiological	Psychological	Sociological
Fluids	Need to maintain necessary fluid intake orally and intra-venously	Parents may not wish further intravenous fluids to be given because of extravasation	
Aeration	Necrotic tissue to be removed to facilitate healing of wound	Parents need to understand *how* and *why* necrotic tissue is removed	
Nutrition	Bottle feeds need to be intro-duced	Parents frightened to feed baby owing to illness	Mother unsure how to feed baby
Communication	Doctors and nurses need to explain implications of injury Documentation essential	Parents frightened and/or angry at hospital, doctors and nurses as to why this injury occurred	Parents may consider legal action against hospital
Activity	Baby needs to be cuddled and handled normally Left foot needs to regain normal movement		Parents need to under-stand importance of bonding
Pain	Dressings chosen that minimize pain on removal Do not restrict movement of foot	Nurses and parents frightened to change dressings if causing Samantha distress and pain	

Histiocytosis X

Histiocytosis X is a rare congenital disorder. The case described in Case Study 4.2 illustrates the problems of managing perineal wounds in babies.

AETIOLOGY
Congenital Abnormalities

Anatomical defects present at birth are classified as congenital abnormalities. This includes, but is not lim-ited to, hereditary disorders.

Congenital abnormalities occur for several reasons. They can be inherited, caused by an embryological defect or can be idiopathic. About 1 in 100 babies is born with a severe malformation, accounting for 1 in 5 stillbirths and 1 in 10 infant deaths.

Histiocytosis X

Histiocytosis X is an extremely rare disorder that affects mainly children under the age of 2 years. The disorder derives its name from the type of body cell involved, the histiocyte (macrophage), with *-osis* meaning increased numbers and X denoting that the cause is unknown.

Case Study 4.2

Histiocytosis

Simon James had been a healthy, normal baby until he was 5 months old, when he developed a generalized rash. This was initially diagnosed as eczema and treated by his general practitioner with emollients and steroid creams, both of which had little effect.

He was referred to a dermatologist, who admitted him to hospital for further investigation and treatment. Skin biopsies of the rash revealed a diagnosis of Langerhans' cell histiocytosis X. Within 5 days of admission Simon's condition deteriorated and he required artificial ventila-tion owing to respiratory distress. In conjunction with his general deterioration, Simon's rash had broken down and ulcerated, with large areas of necrotic eschar cover-ing his abdomen and perineum (Fig. 4.2). The perineal area was also contaminated with urine and faeces and the staff of the paediatric intensive care unit were having trouble keeping a dressing on such a small infant.

Simon's mother was a single parent and lived in poor social circumstances. She had limited understanding of the severity of her son's condition and found it distressing to see his wound dressings being changed, as often they would stick to the skin, causing Simon to cry.

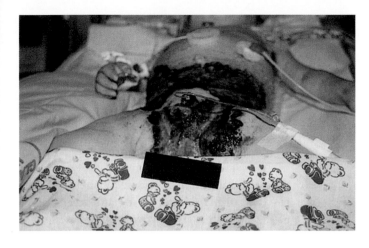

Fig. 4.2 Simon with a large necrotic area on the groin and abdomen.

There are two main types of histiocytosis X; single system and multisystem. In single-system histiocytosis X only one organ in the body is affected, whereas in multisystem disease more than one organ is involved. This disorder is often confused with malignant disease; histiocytosis X is not a type of cancer. The histiocytes do not multiply in situ in an unorganized way but tend to migrate to a site in abnormal numbers or stray outside their normal tissue compartment. Children with histiocytosis X have a deficiency of a certain type of white blood cell, the suppressor lymphocyte.[24]

Prognosis varies. A high incidence of spontaneous remission occurs in single-system disease. Although patients with multisystem disease may spontaneously remit, these children often need treatment. Generally, the younger the child when diagnosed and the more organs involved, the poorer the prognosis. When histiocytosis is diagnosed in older children the disease often runs a more chronic course and may not be life-threatening, although there is associated morbidity, leaving the child with chronic problems.

MANAGEMENT

Managing a wound in the perineum is a difficult nursing problem. Faecal and urinary contamination in a young infant with no bladder or bowel control is inevitable. Frequent wound hygiene is required to keep the bacterial count as low as possible, in combination with dressings and creams that are easily and quickly changed. Skincare including regular washing of the affected parts is essential. The use of an alginate hydrogel or a skin protection cream for the nappy area is recommended. In considering the most appropriate dressing, several points need to be considered:

- Pain and distress are avoided using alginate hydrogel dressings.
- Hydrogels are quickly and easily removed when changing a nappy.
- The treatment is effective (Fig. 4.3).

Nursing Model for Simon

Simon was a previously well infant; both he and his mother now have to *adapt* to the changes in his health status. A model that views the nursing role in terms of supporting patients and their families to adapt to health changes, including illness and its changing demands, through becoming aware of and managing stressors is Roy's adaptation model[25] (see Chapter 2), which can be used to plan Simon's care as shown in Tables 4.2 and 4.3.

Practice Points

- The emphasis of this care plan is placed on minimizing the trauma of being nursed in a 'high technology' area.
- The mother should be involved in Simon's care but only when and if she desires it.
- Her distress at the dressing changes is possibly the way in which she expresses her general anxiety about his overall condition. However, it is one area of care in which she could be involved, provided she has adequate support and guidance.

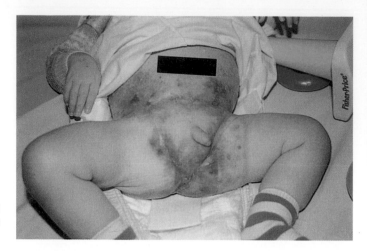

Fig. 4.3 Simon following wound debridement with hydrogel and hydrocellular dressings. The dressings have been held in place with his nappy.

TABLE 4.2 Use of Roy's Adaptation Model to Assess Simon's Care

Life Area	Assessment Level 1 – Behaviour	ASSESSMENT LEVEL 2 – STIMULI		
		Focal	Contextual	Residual
Physiological				
Nutrition	Not taking food orally	Unconscious		
Elimination	No bladder or bowel control	Not yet learnt	Physiological development	
Oxygenation regulation	Unable to breathe spontaneously	Disease process	Mechanical ventilation	
	Necrotic wound areas over perineum and abdomen	Disease process		Rash previously undiagnosed
	Dressings not staying in place	Difficult area to dress	Inexperience of staff dealing with wound	
	Wound contamination	Bladder and bowel incontinence	No continence aids in use	
	Infection of wounds	Cross-contamination from staff Immunosuppressed by disease	High-risk hospital area	
Rest and exercise				
	Normal activity stopped Nursed in frightening environment	Sudden onset of illness	Intensive therapy unit setting	
Self-concept				
	No familiar surroundings to lessen anxiety		Hospital surroundings	Never been in hospital
	Mother unable to understand severity of condition	Sudden onset of illness	Lack of intellectual skills	

TABLE 4.2 Use of Roy's Adaptation Model to Assess Simon's Care—Cont'd

Life Area	Assessment Level 1 – Behaviour	ASSESSMENT LEVEL 2 – STIMULI		
		Focal	Contextual	Residual
Role function				
	Mother unable to provide care, loss of mother role	Mother excluded from care	Lack of social skills to cope	
Interdependency				
	Dependent on staff to provide care	Child too ill, needs specialist staff		No previous experience in hospital
	Mother feels helpless		No support from family, single mother	No previous experience in hospital
	Mother distressed at dressing changes	Not always present when dressings done	Lack of understanding of dressing procedure	No previous hospital experience

TABLE 4.3 Care Plan for Simon

Problem	Goal	Intervention
Unable to breathe spontaneously (A)	Restore oxygenation to normal level	Artificial ventilation
Lack of nutrition (A)	Provide normal nutrition	Intravenous nutrition (check)
Wound contamination from urine (A)	Prevention of urinary incontinence soiling wound	Indwelling catheterization until wound healed
Large amount of necrotic tissue over perineum and abdomen (A)	Removal of necrotic tissue to facilitate healing	Daily application of hydrogel to promote autolysis
Contamination of wound with faeces (A)	Removal of faeces from wound site	Highly absorbent hydrocellular dressing (Allevyn) to remove excess faecal fluid from wound site
Dressings not staying in place	Secure with baby's nappy over dressing	Minimize disturbance of Allevyn sheet
Wound infection (P)	Prevent introduction of infection	Strict asepsis when dressing wound Hand-washing between contacts and when handling soiled nappies
Lack of normal environment (A)	Minimize fear of environment	Staff always to talk, touch and smile with baby Avoid excess use of alarm systems on machines Keep familiar toys and pictures around bed area
Loss of role for mother	Promote mother's involvement	Include mother in care where possible Explain to her why particular treatments are carried out Encourage her to talk to and touch baby
Mother unable to understand severity of condition	Explain in clear terms child's prognosis	Doctors and nurses to use non-medical terms to explain condition Inform mother of changes Do not talk 'over' mother, always with her Involve social worker/health visitor to assess home conditions

Continued

TABLE 4.3	Care Plan for Simon—Cont'd	
Problem	**Goal**	**Intervention**
Mother anxious at surroundings	Minimize her anxiety level	Encourage mother to voice fears to staff Allow time alone with baby if requested Allow time for her to ask questions
Mother distressed at dressing changes	Ensure pain-free dressing changes	Change dressings daily Soak dressings off if signs of adherence Allow mother to help if desired Explain nature and action of dressing products

A, Actual problem; P, potential problem.

Infectious Diseases

One of the most serious infectious diseases in small children is meningitis, as described in Case Study 4.3.

EPIDEMIOLOGY

Although the risk of contracting meningitis is very small, infection rates are highest in children under the age of 5 years, in whom meningococcal infection can cause severe illness very quickly.[26,27] Despite the numerous medical advances that have taken place in paediatrics, the mortality and morbidity rates from meningitis have not decreased. Babies are at higher risk of getting meningitis because they do not have fully developed immune systems; those born earlier than 33 weeks and those weighing less than 2000 g are more at risk.[28] Almost 10% of affected children die and permanent defects affect over 30% of the survivors. The incidence of bacterial meningitis is highest in the first 12 months following birth, with the rates falling as childhood progresses.

AETIOLOGY

Meningitis is inflammation of the meninges, the membranes covering the brain and spinal cord.[29] Bacterial meningitis is an acute, life-threatening infection that requires early diagnosis and appropriate treatment if the patient is to stand the best chance of survival.[30] There is a decline in the incidence of bacterial meningitis in children, thought to be due to the introduction of immunization programmes since the 1980s.[26,30] Organisms causing meningitis vary; interestingly, different pathogens affect specific age groups:

- neonates: group B streptococci, coliform bacteria
- 1 month onwards: *Haemophilus influenzae, Neisseria meningitidis, Streptococcus pneumoniae*
- 1–4 years: *Haemophilus influenzae.*

Case Study 4.3

Infectious Diseases

Lisa Evans, a previously healthy 11-month-old child, had been ill for a week with a cold, cough and sore throat.

Her condition deteriorated one evening when she became very hot and began to vomit. Following three episodes of vomiting she became listless and appeared to be losing consciousness. Her mother called the general practitioner who arranged her immediate admission to hospital with suspected meningococcal meningitis.

Following admission, Lisa was transferred to the intensive care unit for intubation and intravenous antibiotic therapy. By the following day she had developed a purpuric rash over her trunk, buttocks and legs and she was diagnosed as having meningococcal septicaemia.

Within the next 3 days the purpuric rash had spread (Fig. 4.4) to involve both arms and was blistering, necrotic and wet. Lisa had responded well to her antibiotics and was breathing spontaneously but continued to be nursed in a high-dependency area off the intensive care unit.

Diagnosis of meningitis is difficult, with symptoms being vague and, in the first instance, identical to many other, less dangerous, childhood illnesses. Typically the infant will develop a generalized febrile illness with unusual irritability or lethargy.[11] This rapidly develops to include other symptoms such as vomiting and seizures as the infant's condition deteriorates. Nuchal rigidity or a bulging fontanelle occurs in less than 50% of infants and small children.[27] The purpuric rash of meningococcal meningitis is associated with an overwhelming infection with Gram-negative diplococci or meningococci, causing haemorrhage

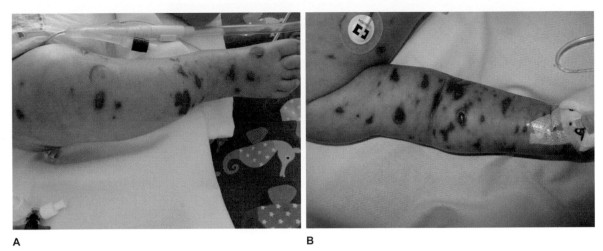

A   **B**

Fig. 4.4 Purpuric rash of meningococcal meningitis on legs (A) and on arm (B) in 11-month-old infant Lisa.

through toxic damage to the capillaries. Skin damage from this rash can often be so severe that full-thickness skin loss and ulceration result in permanent damage. Other long-term complications include hearing loss, seizures and learning difficulties.[27]

Diagnosis is based on:

- the presence of a non-specific febrile illness
- raised intracranial pressure, clinical signs of which include reduced and declining level of consciousness, extensor hypertonia, cranial nerve palsy, dilated pupils, bradycardia and high blood pressure
- positive blood culture
- lumbar puncture to obtain cerebrospinal fluid, which will demonstrate raised levels of white cells and protein and reduced glucose concentration.

MANAGEMENT

Patient outcome is dependent on early diagnosis and treatment. Third-generation cephalosporins offer a safer and more effective alternative to the previously popular antibiotic regimens of chloramphenicol and penicillins. However, there is an increasing resistance of bacteria to some antibiotics.[27] These infants are best nursed on paediatric intensive care units with aggressive support of cardiovascular function, elective ventilation and measures to reduce raised intracranial pressure. If the infant survives this acute stage of the illness, bacterial toxins can cause other problems such as vascular damage.

Ulceration can be treated with excision and grafting, a process that will hasten healing but will depend on the child's general condition and the availability of plastic surgery. Wounds in these children have to be treated by an experienced paediatric plastic surgery team, for example at a paediatric burns unit, and need surgical performance for best outcome. Amputation of body parts may be necessary.

Nursing Model for Lisa

Lisa's condition is life-threatening and although the nurse needs to establish a good relationship with the parents, her first priority will be assessing Lisa's physical condition.

The correct management of the child's wound at this stage may avoid or minimize the scarring that could result from her meningococcal rash. Using Peplau's model, assess Lisa's needs under the SOAP structure (see Chapter 2).[31]

S – *subjective* feelings and experiences of the patient or parent

O – *objective* observation by nurse

A – formal *assessment* and identification of the problem

P – *plan* of action.

For example, with regard to the wound:

S: Mother is concerned at the large amount of 'black scabs' on wound.

O: There are large areas of necrotic tissue preventing wound from healing.

A: Problem statement or goal: necrotic tissue requires removal.

P: Plan:

Apply hydrogel to facilitate autolysis.

Apply low-adherent dressings.

With regard to the psychosocial aspect of the situation:

S: Mother is anxious that Lisa will not recover from meningitis.

O: Vital signs are now within normal limits and baby is recovering:

Baby is breathing spontaneously.

Baby displays no signs of cerebral irritation.

A: Mother's anxiety level high; she needs support and information.

P: Provide mother with information and reassurance of baby's recovery:

Encourage mother to stay with baby.

Inform mother of changes in baby's condition.

Encourage mother to participate in baby's care.

Practice Points

- Observations could also be made concerned with recording the wound size, ensuring wounds do not become macerated and that removal of the dressings is painless for the baby.
- The mother will need advice regarding how long treatment of her baby's wounds may take and how she can help care for Lisa during this period.

Thermal Injuries

Wounds from burns and scalds in young children are frequently encountered in nursing practice. An example of an accidental injury of this type is given in Case Study 4.4.

EPIDEMIOLOGY

Thermal injuries from flame, burns and scalds are extremely common in young children. In the UK 125,000 children require hospital treatment each year for these injuries,[32] of whom about 50% have been injured in the kitchen following scalds from hot liquids. Hot drinks are involved in about 1265 of severe burns, 1100 of these occurring in children under 5 years of age. Lawrence and Carson[33] tracked the

---

Case Study 4.4

Thermal Injuries

Lucy Llewellyn was just 2 years old when she was admitted to Primrose Ward one morning as an emergency. Lucy, the youngest of three children, had gone into the kitchen unsupervised that morning and reached up to the kitchen unit to get her teddy bear. Unfortunately she had not seen the full cup of tea her father had left just on the edge and tipped it over herself, scalding her shoulder, upper arm and chest. Her mother, alerted by Lucy's screams, had the foresight to immediately remove the clothing and run the scalded areas under the tap for 10 minutes, and cover the area with a clean tea towel. The father called an ambulance that took her to the local hospital where Lucy was treated for a deep, partial-thickness injury to her shoulder and upper arm and a superficial partial-thickness injury to her chest. Although these injuries were serious, the mother's quick action had prevented further damage (Fig. 4.5).

---

increase in kettle scalds since the 1920s and report that a marked increase in this injury is related to the introduction of plastic jug kettles.

MANAGEMENT

Correct and prompt first aid management of burns and scalds can substantially reduce the depth of tissue damage. Immediate immersion in cold water (not colder than 25°C) for a maximum of 10 minutes rapidly quenches residual heat and eases pain.[34,35] Parents, however, may be distressed at their screaming child, not know how long to apply cold water and be alarmed by seeing skin peel off. It should be stressed that the burn or scald will continue to develop with redness and blistering and appear to enlarge. Seconds are often lost by removal of clothing, which should also be drenched to save time.[36] The burned area will be debrided in a hospital and therefore a special dressing by parents before transmitting the child to hospital/healthcare service is not necessary.

Thermal injuries are classified according to depth.[29]

- *Superficial burn*: presents as erythema or mild erythema and pain. The reddened area blanches with pressure. Occurs following sunburn or flash burn. Heals within 3–7 days with no scarring.

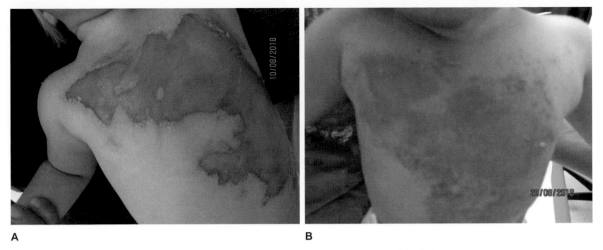

Fig. 4.5 Baby Lucy showing (A) acute wounds; (B) wounds healed.

- *Partial-thickness skin loss*: fluid lost from the burn wound either forms blisters under damaged skin or exudate from areas where the outer layers have been lost.
  - *Superficial partial-thickness skin loss*: the epidermis and superficial layers of the dermis are destroyed. Hair follicles, sebaceous and sweat glands are, however, spared. From these epithelial structures, migration of cells rapidly occurs to provide an intact surface within 10–21 days. Pain is experienced when the nerve endings of the dermis have not been damaged. The wound usually heals without scarring.
  - *Deep partial-thickness skin loss*: a greater part of the dermis is lost and little of the skin appendages remain. Healing is delayed. Sensation is altered – patient has blunting of pinprick sensation.
- *Full-thickness skin loss*: there are no surviving epithelial elements in full-thickness loss. The burn can only heal by contraction and by migration of existing epithelial cells at the edges of the wound. The wound may look pale and charred and coagulated veins may be visible. No sensation is present on testing.

Nursing the Child Following Injury

On admission to the children's ward an initial assessment of the child will take into account that the child has not been prepared for admission and may be very frightened. As a result the child may be fractious, crying and clinging to his/her parents. Often parents experience feelings of guilt for not protecting the child from the accident. Children with severe burns should be transmitted to specialized paediatric burns centres (https://www.euroburn.org/burn-centres/). On admission the nurse will aim to:

- use a calm and friendly approach to the child and family to comfort and reassure the child. The child will be assured that her mother or father will be able to stay with her so that she will not be left alone
- encourage the parents to cuddle and care for the child. Intravenous infusions and other equipment need not prevent parents from maintaining close contact with their child
- explain to the child and parents, using terms they will understand, any procedures that may need to be performed
- be non-judgemental, to reassure the parents that blame is not being apportioned. Some parents may want to talk about the accident and may be obviously distressed. The nurse will aim to restore the parents' confidence and self-esteem as they may be feeling inadequate and guilty.

Longer-term aims of the nursing care are:

- to help the parents understand that their child may take time in adapting to the new environment and that behavioural disturbances are to be expected.[17] Their child may become aggressive and difficult or, alternatively, may become quiet and withdrawn. Behavioural regression may take many forms and parents need the reassurance that this is temporary

- to encourage the child to become independent again and restore her self-confidence
- to introduce the child to play leaders, nursery nurses and teachers, where appropriate, to minimize boredom. Television, videos and computer games can also help with this.

Over a period of time the nurse may be able to take on a health educator role in helping the parents to understand how the accident happened and how it may be prevented in the future. This involves looking at a number of factors contributing to the accident and including the child, the agent involved (e.g., the cup of tea) and the physical and social context in which the accident happened.

Non-Accidental Injury

In the accident and emergency department parents are likely to be closely questioned on how the accident happened and what action they took subsequently. The child may also be asked what happened, although in Lucy's case this would not be admissible as she is shocked and distressed. Staff will always need to ascertain whether the distribution of injury fits the history given by the parents.

Effects of Hypertrophic Scarring

Unfortunately the hypertrophic scarring following a burn or scald can be a constant disfiguring reminder to the child of the causative accident. Hypertrophic scars are red, firm and thickened and cause intense itching (see Chapter 1).

Although hypertrophic scarring usually flattens as the scar matures, there is evidence that the use of constant, long-term pressure can prevent its formation.[11] Several preventive and treatment options are available for reducing scarring including silicone sheets, pressure garments, chemical peels and vitamin creams.[37] Pressure garments are popular and are used to apply pressure on the torso and limbs and help realignment of the collagen fibres. These are worn for 24 hours daily and removed only for cleansing or bathing for the first 9 months[38] for a period of up to 2 years. Garments will need frequent replacement in the growing child and great care is required to ensure they are comfortable and well fitting. The wearing of such garments can have a profound effect on small children and will affect all sorts of normal activities of a 2-year-old, such as swimming and the wearing of dresses.

Success has also been achieved with topical application of silicone gel sheeting, although its mode of action is unclear. The sheeting is cut to size and secured with adhesive tape and needs to be worn for several weeks, day and night.[39]

Treatment of Burns and Scalds

On admission to an accident and emergency department, a thorough history of the accident will be taken from the parents and/or child.

For major burn injuries or deep skin loss around the face and neck, the main concern is maintenance of a clear airway. The percentage size of the burn is calculated using the Lund and Browder chart (Fig. 4.6). The child's weight is taken and assessment of fluid requirements calculated. If the burn is over 10% of the body surface pain relief and tetanus toxoid will be given where required, depending on the depth and type of burn injury.

Wound Dressings

The burn or scald should be swabbed prior to cleansing, to ascertain the type of bacteria present in the wound. Bacterial colonization of all thermal wounds occurs following injury but generally causes no problems with healing, the greatest risk being cross-contamination between patients.[11] Certain organisms, however, may cause particular problems, especially *Staphylococcus aureus* which can result in toxic shock syndrome.

Cleansing should be performed with saline (see Chapter 3), using irrigation techniques. Dead epithelium and blisters are removed using sterile scissors, with debridement of necrotic material under strict aseptic conditions. Deep dermal burns will require surgical debridement in theatre followed by excision and grafting.

Following cleansing, burns should be covered with a low-adherent dressing. Films and hydrocolloids will provide moist wound healing and protection for superficial burns with low-to-moderate levels of exudate.[34] More heavily exuding wounds can

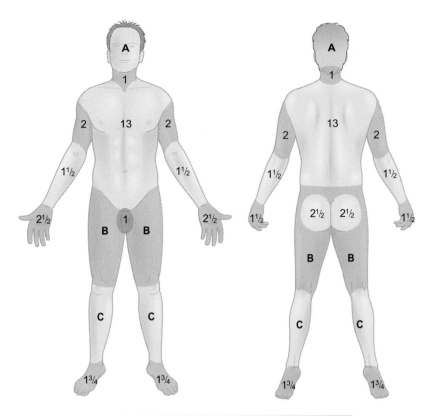

Relative percentage of areas affected by growth						
Age in years	0	1	5	10	15	Adult
A = ½ of head	9½	8½	6½	5½	4½	3½
B = ½ of one thigh	2¾	3¼	3	4¼	4½	4¾
C = ½ of one leg	2½	2½	2¾	3	3¼	3½

Fig. 4.6 Lund and Browder chart. (Reproduced by kind permission of Smith & Nephew Pharmaceuticals.)

be dressed with alginates, foams and hydrofibre dressings. Silver-containing foam dressings are also widely used.

Nursing Model for Lucy

There are many issues at stake for Lucy and her family. The nurse on the ward needs to build a strong, trusting relationship with the toddler and her parents. As with Samantha (Case Study 4.1), it is important to look at psychological and sociological aspects as well as physiological care for Lucy and her parents. Riehl's model is therefore a useful framework for the initial assessment. Look at the problems identified below and consider how you could help the child and her parents. Look at the situation from the parents' and child's points of view.

Physiological (A, actual; P, potential)
- pain due to burn injury (A)
- risk of infection in wound site (P)
- hypertrophic scarring following wound healing (P)
- dressings adhering to wound causing painful dressing change (P)
- child not wanting nurses to change the dressings (P).

Psychological

- parents, particularly father, feeling guilty about accident (A)
- child not understanding what has happened to her (A)
- repeated questioning in accident and emergency department and ward reinforcing feelings of guilt (P).

Sociological

- child suddenly put in unfamiliar surroundings owing to emergency admission (A)
- lack of parental knowledge with regard to prevention of further accidents (A)
- parents separated from other children (A)
- parents labelled by ward staff as uncaring and careless (P)
- child at risk of non-accidental injury (A).

Practice Points

- There are many psychological factors influencing the parents but the child may have psychological effects in the long term, so this should be considered now.
- This case highlights the need for the specialist skills of trained paediatric nurses when dealing

Summary

This chapter has dealt mainly with wounds that have a traumatic aetiology – the most common type of children's wound that nurses have to treat. In children, direct management of the traumatic wound can often appear straightforward. However, when nursing infants and children with wounds, some of the greatest challenges concern the psychological and sociological impact. The models that have been chosen to assess the care in each of the case studies have largely concentrated on these important areas and are not easy options on busy paediatric units. They do, hopefully, encourage the practitioner to think about such issues as:

- communication skills – with child, parents and team members
- legal and moral aspects of care – documentation, non-disclosure of information, choice of treatments
- organizational skills – planned management of care
- dressing choices – alleviation of painful dressing changes, minimization of scarring.

with traumatic injuries in infants. How the care is planned will depend on the experience of the nurse. Inexperienced practitioners may not even identify some of these problems and may not be equipped to provide the required management.

- Think of the specific skills that a nurse requires to deal with this case.

FURTHER READING

Department of Health 2004. *PRODIGY Guidance – Burns and Scalds.* Department of Health; 2004. Infant mortality rates 1976–2003. Available at: www.statistics.gov.uk.

Huband S, Trigg E. *Practices in Children's Nursing.* Edinburgh: Churchill Livingstone; 2000.

Lawrence JC, Cason C. Kettle scalds. *J Wound Care.* 1994;3(6):289–292.

REFERENCES

1. United Nations. *The United Nations Convention on the Rights of the Child.* New York, NY: United Nations. Available at: https://www.unicef.org.uk/what-we-do/un-convention-child-rights/.
2. American Academy of Pediatrics (AAP). *Newborns, Infants, and Toddlers*; 2002. Available at: http://patiented.aap.org/categoryBrowse.aspx?catID=5001.
3. Ciprandi G, Romanelli M, Durante CM, Baharestani M, Meuli M. Both skill and sensitivity are needed for paediatric patients. Guest Editorial. *Wounds Int.* 2012;3(1):5.
4. Department of Health. *Infant, perinatal and neonatal deaths*; 2015. Available at: https://www.ons.gov.uk/peoplepopulationandcommunity/birthsdeathsandmarriages/deaths/bulletins/deathsregistrationsummarytables/2015-07-15.
5. Muscari ME. Pediatric nursing overview. In: *Pediatric Nursing.* Philadelphia: Lippincott; 2001.
6. Blume-Peytavi U, Hauser M, Stamatas GN, Pathirana D, Garcia Bartels N. Skin care practices for newborn and infants: review of the clinical evidence for best practices. *Pediatr Dermatol.* 2012;29:1–14.
7. Nikolovski J, Stamatas GN, Kollias N, Wiegand BC. Barrier function and water-holding and transport properties of infant stratum corneum are different from adult and continue to develop through the first year of life. *J Invest Dermatol.* 2008;128:1728–1736.
8. Stamatas GN, Nikolovski J, Luedtke MA, Kollias N, Wiegand BC. Infant skin microstructure assessed in vivo differs from adult skin in organization and at the cellular level. *Pediatr Dermatol.* 2010;27:125–131.
9. Dellinger RP, Levy MM, Rhodes A, et al. Surviving sepsis campaign: international guidelines for management of severe sepsis and septic shock. *Intensive Care Med.* 2012;39(2013):165–228.
10. MacQueen S. Wound care. In: Huband S, Trigg E, eds. *Practices in Children's Nursing.* Edinburgh: Churchill Livingstone; 2000.
11. Hazinski MF. *Manual of Pediatric Critical Care.* St Louis, Missouri: Mosby; 1999.
12. O'Dwyer J. Introduction to community. In: Huband S, Trigg E, eds. *Practices in Children's Nursing.* Edinburgh: Churchill Livingstone; 2000.
13. Fearon J. Assessment. In: Huband S, Trigg E, eds. *Practices in Children's Nursing.* Edinburgh: Churchill Livingstone; 2000.

14. Kay J. Hygiene. In: Huband S, Trigg E, eds. *Practices in Children's Nursing*. Edinburgh: Churchill Livingstone; 2000.
15. Colson J. Concepts. In: Huband S, Trigg E, eds. *Practices in Children's Nursing*. Edinburgh: Churchill Livingstone; 2000.
16. Teare J. A home care team in paediatric wound care. *J Wound Care*. 1997;6(6):295–296.
17. Butler NR. Perinatal problems. In: Huband S, Trigg E, eds. *Practices in Children's Nursing*. Edinburgh: Churchill Livingstone; 2000.
18. Llewellyn N. Pain assessment and the use of morphine. *Paediatr Nurs*. 1994;6(1):25–30.
19. Bale S, Jones V. The care of children with wounds. *J Wound Care*. 1996;5(4):177–180.
20. Mohammed TA. Venepuncture and cannulation. In: Huband S, Trigg E, eds. *Practices in Children's Nursing*. Edinburgh: Churchill Livingstone; 2000.
21. Young T. Wound healing in neonates. *J Wound Care*. 1995;4(6):285–288.
22. Riehl-Sisca JP. The Riehl interaction model. In: Riehl-Sisca JP, ed. *Conceptual Models for Nursing Practice*. 3rd ed. Norwalk: Connecticut: Appleton and Lange; 1989.
23. Abbey J. The FANCAP assessment scheme. In: Riehl JP, Roy C, eds. *Conceptual Models for Nursing Practice*. New York: Appleton-Century-Crofts; 1980.
24. Riggs RL, Bale S. Management of necrotic wounds as a complication of histiocytosis X. *J Wound Care*. 1993;2(5):260–261.
25. Roy C, Andrews H. *The Roy Adaptation Model*. 2nd ed. Stamford: Connecticut: Appleton and Lange; 1999.
26. Hederman RS, Lambert HP, O'Sullivan I, Stuart JM, Taylor BL, Wall RA. Early management of suspected bacterial meningitis and meningococcal septaemia in Adults. *J Hosp Infect*. 2003;46:75–77.
27. Phillips EJ, Simor AE. Bacterial meningitis in children and adults. *Postgrad Med*. 1998;103(3):116–129.
28. Meningitis Research Foundation. Meningococcal disease; 2002. Available at: www.meningitis.org.
29. Phipps A. Evidence based management of patients with burns. *J Wound Care*. 1998;7(6):299–302.
30. Spach DH. New issues in bacterial meningitis in adults. *Postgrad Med*. 2003;114(5):65–74.
31. Peplau H. *Interpersonal Relations in Nursing*. New York: G P Putman; 1952.
32. National Burns Care Review Committee. *National Burn Care Review*. British Association of Plastic Surgeons; 2001. Available at: www.baps.co.uk.
33. Lawrence JC, Carson C. Kettle scalds. *J Wound Care*. 1994;3(6):289–292.
34. Dowsett C. The assessment and management of burns. *Br J Community Nurs*. 2002;7(5):230–239.
35. McCormack A, La Hei ER, Martin HC. First-aid management of minor burns in children: a prospective study of children presenting to the Children's Hospital at Westmead, Sydney. *Med J Aust*. 2003;178(1):31–33.
36. Mertens DM, Jenkins M, Warden G. Outpatient burns management. *Nurs Clin North Am*. 1997;32(2):343–364.
37. O'Kane S. Wound remodelling and scarring. *J Wound Care*. 2002;11(8):296–299.
38. Pape SA. The management of scars. *J Wound Care*. 1993;2(6):354–360.
39. SMTL. SMTL data card for dressing silicone sheet; 2004. Available at: www.dressings.org.

MCQS

1 *What is most appropriate choice of wound dressing for neonates and infants?*
a. One that the baby likes the colour of
b. One that fits easily to the wound
c. One that avoids further harm to the fragile skin around the defect area
d. One that is cheap because wounds in children need to be changed more frequently

2 *Burns and scalds are common injuries in children. How long should family, parents or the emergency team cool the affected area?*
a. For more than 15 minutes with cold water
b. For a few minutes with water containing ice cubes
c. For 10 minutes using gel or oil for cooling
d. For a maximum of 10 minutes using water no colder than 25°C.

3 *How should parents be advised with regard to visiting when a neonate is cared for in hospital?*
a. To be with their child as much as possible
b. To only stay for a few hours each day to limit their stress
c. To support nursing care as much as they want and feel confident to
d. To spend every second day with their child so as to avoid long separation

Chapter 5

Wound Care in Teenagers

Anna-Barbara Schlüer

Highlights

As you read through this chapter concentrate on the following.

- inadequate wound management that may affect the rest of the teenager's life
- aspects of privacy, body image and personal identity important to a teenager
- emotional effects that injury may have on the teenager
- devastating effect of disablement or disfigurement on the rest of the teenager's life.

Key Issues

This chapter outlines the most common wound problems encountered by the teenager.

Clinical Case Studies

Aetiology and management of:

- A young boy sustaining chemical burns caused by battery acid
- Pressure sore in a young girl with spina bifida
- Traumatic injuries due to a road traffic accident

Nursing Models

Examples of their application to practice are taken from:

- Roper's activities of living model
- Orem's model
- Roy's adaptation model

Introduction

Of all the phases of the life cycle, adolescence is undoubtedly one of the most difficult. During the adolescent period the individual changes from a child into an adult and strives to achieve social and emotional maturity. The duration of adolescence and the age at which it occurs is difficult to determine, as each individual varies. Adolescence has been defined as a phase of physiological, physical and psychological change through which an individual progresses to reach maturity.[1,2] Body image issues dominate as peers set standards for appearance and behaviour and peer group pressure is strong. Being accepted by peers is a fundamental issue for youths and at this age individuals may set out to impress others by acting irresponsibly and taking unnecessary risks. Concerns about illness may focus on changes in physical appearance that might not be deemed acceptable by peers.

Common behavioural traits exhibited by adolescents include mood swings, rebellion, periodic regression, self-preoccupation and antagonism. Coming to terms with the adult world can be an extremely traumatic time for the young individual. Illness and hospitalization of adolescents can be difficult when often their physical needs take precedence over their emotional needs. Health professionals, including nurses, need to be very aware of the needs and rights of teenagers, especially when considering their independence, privacy and social needs.[1,3] Adolescent wards allow teenagers to be cared for in specialized units designed to meet their specific needs. Such needs include body image and personal identity issues, independence (social and financial) from parents and help in communicating and developing social skills.[2]

Specific problems for adolescents being treated in hospital[3] include:

- lack of privacy
- problems associated with change of body image and loss of self-worth
- anxiety related to hospitalization
- regression

Chemical Burns (Fig. 5.1)

David Oskim, a 17-year-old schoolboy, has always had a keen interest in cars and car maintenance. Last month he secured a Saturday job in the local garage as a trainee mechanic. He was particularly pleased as his father had just bought him a car and he was having driving lessons.

The garage owner was pleased to take David on because of his enthusiasm but also because he only needed to pay him a small amount of money. A hard-working, conscientious man, he had little time to give David a proper induction and assumed David was aware of the usual hazards of working in this environment.

One Saturday David was working on an engine that required him to remove and drain the battery. While lifting the battery out of its casing, David let it slip and tipped battery acid over his forearm. The owner, who had not experienced this type of accident before, immediately led David to the washbasin, plunged his arm and hand in a basin of cold water and removed the sleeve of his overall. While telephoning for an ambulance, he told David to keep his arm under the tap. On arrival at the accident and emergency department David was shocked and in a great deal of pain, having sustained a superficial partial-thickness burn to his forearm.

- restriction of normal physical activities
- fear of death in the seriously ill
- loss of independence.

The adolescent period is one in which accidental and traumatic injuries are common and both mortality and morbidity rates are high. Wounds frequently result from such injuries. In 2014, 25% of deaths among young people aged 15-19 in Europe were caused by transport accidents.[4]

After injuries, leading causes of death for adolescents include cancer, heart disease and birth defects. When it comes to wound management in this age group, choice of dressings and wound treatment are in line with adult wound care.

Chemical Burns

Case Study 5.1 illustrates the case of a schoolboy injured in an industrial accident with corrosive materials.

TABLE 5.1 First Aid Received by a Selection of Patients Admitted to a Burns Unit

Patient Group	FIRST AID RECEIVED		
	Satisfactory	Unsatisfactory	None
Children	15	3	6
Adults at home	9	3	10
Industrial cases	7	3	8
Other cases not in or around the home	2	3	2
Total	33	12	26

Reproduced with kind permission from Petch N, Cason CG. Examining first aid received by burn and scald patients. *Journal of Wound Care*. 1993;2(2):102–105.

AETIOLOGY

Industrial accidents continue to be part of everyday working life. In the UK fatal accidents are decreasing from 179 in 2008 tzo 147 in 2018.[5] From a workforce of one thousand, 75 workers suffered from a burn or scald at work.[6]

The level of first aid these workers receive will greatly affect their prognosis and degree of injury. In a study undertaken by Petch and Cason,[7] of the first aid received by 18 patients admitted to a burns unit as a result of industrial accident, only seven had received satisfactory first aid, while eight had received none at all (Table 5.1).

MANAGEMENT

The rapid removal of corrosive chemicals from the skin is an urgent first aid requirement. Highly acid and alkaline substances are readily absorbed into the tissues, causing rapid burning to the affected area (Fig. 5.1). Irrigation of the burnt area with copious quantities of water should normally be commenced as soon as possible, with some exceptions. Any clothing in contact with the injured area should be cut away and the skin irrigation continued until an ambulance arrives or *en route* to the accident and emergency department.[8] Full details of the nature and composition of the corrosive chemical causing the burn will be needed by the hospital, so every attempt should be made to identify the substance. Some chemicals have specific antidotes that can be given in the

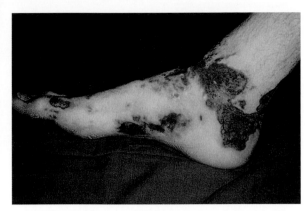

Fig. 5.1 Chemical burn. (Reproduced with kind permission of Jan Olsen, Burns Unit, Morriston Hospital, Swansea.)

accident and emergency department. It is important to note that not all chemical burns should be irrigated with water. Substances containing metallic sodium, potassium and lithium should not be irrigated with water.[9,10]

In hospital an assessment of the degree and extent of the burns will be made. The Lund and Browder chart (see Fig. 4.6) is now considered to be a more effective method of assessing extent of burns injuries than the 'rule of nine'.[1]

The depth of burn should be assessed and recorded. This can be done by estimating the loss of epidermis, dermis and appendages (see Chapter 4).

Treatment of small burns may be carried out in the accident and emergency department without the need to admit the young person. Debridement of devitalized tissue is essential. Where surgical debridement is needed to remove devitalized tissue, the hospital stay may be only a few days. The use of modern wound dressings for full-thickness burns is applicable where infection has been eliminated so that daily activity is relatively unaffected. Hydrogels, foams and alginates may all have a role to play.

- Hydrogels are comfortable and conformable, provide moisture at the wound bed and can be used with semipermeable films, thus allowing bathing, etc.
- Foams are comfortable and absorbent and some are adhesive.
- Alginates are absorbent and comfortable and can be used with pads or semipermeable films to allow bathing, etc.

Returning to normal activities, such as swimming and sports, may be facilitated by using occlusive dressings. Monitoring of the healing wound may be undertaken by the practice or district nurse in conjunction with the parents, although teenagers may wish to care for their own wounds on a day-to-day basis. Tetanus protection is essential for all types of burns, irrespective of depth. The choice of dressing material will depend on a thorough assessment of the patient, and the lifestyle of the adolescent will need to be taken into consideration.

The long-term consequences of a chemical burn may be disfiguring, with scarring of the affected area. The adolescent and parents may wish to take legal action against the employer if negligence is involved. The Health and Safety Act may be invoked to prevent recurrence of such an accident and procedures for handling chemicals may need to be reviewed.

Nursing Model for David

Luckily for David, his employer took the right course of first aid action, although he should have ensured David had adequate Health and Safety advice before he took the job.

Although a partial-thickness burn should heal without scarring, the type of care David receives now may influence the rest of his life. Any injury to a hand, however superficial, should ideally be assessed by a plastic surgeon.

Roper's model[11] has been used to assess David's care (Table 5.2). The assessment reveals that David has the following major problems:

Motor Activities
- cannot wash
- cannot eat normally
- cannot work
- cannot write
- cannot drive
- pain.

Psychosocial Aspects
- disruption in schooling/workplace
- anxiety
- self-image (effect of scarring).

TABLE 5.2	Assessment of David's Problems (Case Study 5.1)
Activities of Living	**Problem Statements**
Eliminating	Normal bowel action
	Normal urine output
	Cannot use right hand to attend to personal hygiene following elimination
Eating and drinking	Good diet and fluid intake but cannot eat very well with one hand
Working and play-ing	Unable to continue work, cannot write as right-handed
	Future employment/education may be affected
	Just started driving lessons which he cannot continue
Sleeping	Arm and hand still quite painful, cannot get comfortable at night
	Worried about employment and school work
Personal cleansing	Cannot wash or shower very well
Expressing sexuality	Worried about effects of burns or scarring to his arm and hand

Practice Points

For an apparently small injury there are many complications:

- The management of the burnt hand can best be achieved with silver sulphadiazine in a sterile plastic bag; the arm can be covered with a film dressing or other low-adherent material. Neither arm nor hand will require grafting.
- Documentation of treatment and wound assessment must be meticulous in case there are complications at a later date.
- Think about how this accident could have been avoided.

Pressure Ulcers

Pressure ulcers are normally associated with elderly patients but can occur in young patients with disabilities such as spina bifida, as discussed in Case Study 5.2.

Case Study 5.2

Pressure Ulcers in a Physically Disabled Teenager

Thirteen-year-old Tracy Childs was born with spina bifida and has been paralysed from the waist down since birth. Incontinent of faeces and urine, Tracy has been hospitalized many times for urinary diversion and now has a permanent urostomy.

Tracy lives with her mother and father and younger brother John, who is 7 years old. The family house has been adapted for Tracy's wheelchair and has a downstairs bathroom with shower. Although dogged by episodes of ill health, Tracy remains a cheerful and determined teenager that, with her devoted mother giving 24-hour care, copes well with her disabilities.

Six weeks ago Tracy complained of feeling unwell and was diagnosed as having a urinary infection. Despite a course of oral antibiotics she became nauseated and confused and had a temperature of 40°C. She was rushed into hospital where she received intravenous antibiotics and for several days was seriously ill. Unable to eat food, she lost 4.5 kg in weight. Because of her position in bed and lack of her usual stoma bags, urine leaked out around her conduit. This resulted on three occasions in Tracy lying in one position for several hours on wet sheets. When she finally became well she was put in an ordinary wheelchair without the pressure-relieving cushion that she would normally have in her wheelchair at home.

Tracy's mother was distressed at the apparent lack of attention to her daughter's needs. Although the staff were caring, the ward was obviously inadequately staffed and lacked what Tracy's mother viewed as essential equipment. On her mother's insistence, Tracy was discharged home as soon as her temperature became normal and prescribed an oral antibiotic regimen. The day after discharge, in the course of a blanket bath, Tracy's mother noticed two broken areas of skin on the teenager's left hip and right ischial tuberosity. Two days later they became black in the middle and deep red around the outside (Fig. 5.2). She was horrified, realizing these were pressure ulcers, and called the GP, who sent the district nurse to assess the situation.

AETIOLOGY

Spina bifida is caused by defective closure of the caudal neuropore towards the end of the fourth week of gestation. Spina bifida occulta (non-fusion of the spinal arches limited to vertebral defects) occurs in around 10% of the population. Although a small

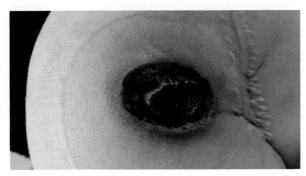

Fig. 5.2 Teenager with spina bifida with a deep undermining pressure ulcer.

dimple or hair tuft can be seen, individuals are generally asymptomatic. However, spina bifida cystica is less common, occurring in 1 in 1000 births. The lesion is sac-like in appearance, with multiple unfused vertebrae. The lesions can be closed, with either the meninges alone (meningocele) or both the meninges and the spinal cord (meningomyelocele) within the sac. A more severe version, myeloschisis, occurs when an open neural tube is present without an overlying sac. Spina bifida causes severe neurological defects corresponding to the level at which the defect is found.[12]

Children born with high lesions have a poor neurological prognosis and the majority of patients experience both bladder and bowel problems. For children with meningomyelocele, a common complication is hydrocephalus. Owing to their immobility, it is not unusual for these individuals to have many episodes of pressure ulcers (Fig. 5.2).

MANAGEMENT

The management of pressure ulcers in children or teenagers with chronic illness or disability needs to address four important issues:

- maintenance of self-care and independence
- provision of pressure-relieving and other equipment such as wheelchairs
- implications of pressure ulcers on the patient's general health and disability
- prevention on any further skin breakdown or pressure issue to the skin.

It needs to be stressed that the effect of having a pressure ulcer will alter the whole lifestyle of the individual. Also the likelihood of further breakdown increases if adequate preventive measures are not put in place as a permanent part of management.

Multiple ulcer development over a period of time will cause further disability, require plastic surgery and predispose to life-threatening systemic infections.

The management of category IV necrotic pressure ulcers is particularly problematic, as the extent of the tissue damage under the necrotic eschar is often hidden. Damage may be superficial or may extend down to muscle and bone. This is a serious and potentially hazardous situation for a patient where severe and deep-seated infection causes septicaemia and organ failure. Debridement of this devitalized necrotic tissue can be achieved in several ways – surgically, chemically and by autolysis using dressings (see Chapter 8). Tracy may choose a conservative method of treatment that can be carried out at home by the district nurse. A hydrogel used with a semipermeable film in conjunction with sharp debridement of loose devitalized tissue is a common form of treatment. Negative-pressure wound treatment can be successful once the necrotic tissue is removed.

For chair-bound individuals, a written plan for the use of repositioning devices, negotiated between the individual and the professionals and tailored to the specific needs of the individual, is an effective way of reducing the likelihood of pressure ulcers.[13] Included in this type of plan would be consideration of postural alignment, distribution of weight, balance and stability, and pressure relief.

A seat cushion is essential for providing pressure relief in wheelchairs, as very high pressures can be exerted by wheelchair base seats.[14] In addition to using an appropriate seat cushion, chair-bound individuals can be taught to relieve presssssure by shifting their weight regularly throughout the day. Relief of the high levels of pressure produced by sitting should be undertaken at least hourly. For patients with spinal cord injuries, weight shifts have been shown to be effective in reducing the risk of pressure ulcers.[15]

The care and management outlined below can be used as a framework for many individuals in similar situations.

Nursing Model for Tracy

When assessing and planning Tracy's care, the district nurse must be fully aware of Tracy's previous history. The nurse must also assess the family as a unit and not consider Tracy's needs apart from her family. Also, as a

TABLE 5.3	Assessment of Tracy (Case Study 5.2) Using Orem's Model	
Self-Care Need	**Self-Care Ability**	**Self-Care Deficit**
Sufficient intake of air	Tracy breathes without problems whichever position she is placed in	Nil
Fluid balance	Tracy is required to drink 2–3 L daily to keep kidneys patent feels weak following hospitalization	Needs extra fluids (A) Further urinary tract infection (P) Renal failure (P)
Nutrition	Extra energy needed owing to pressure ulcers and weight loss tracy has never had a large appetite	Weight loss (A) Catabolic state (A) Poor diet (A)
Elimination	Urostomy bag leaking due to weight loss and lying in bed bowels evacuated daily by manual evacuation	Cannot manage urostomy without leakage (A) Diarrhoea due to antibiotics (P) Increased interface friction (P)
Activity and rest	Has had prolonged period in bed Will continue to spend more time in bed, not in wheelchair, owing to pressure ulcers	Inadequate exercise (A) Muscle wasting (P) Non-healing pressure ulcers (A) Further skin breakdown (P)
Socializing	Normally a very sociable girl, Tracy has had a long period in hospital without her usual social contacts Mother has spent long periods in hospital with her	Depressed due to enforced hospitalization (A)
Normalcy	Normally goes to school, has family outings and friends to the house considers her disability as normal to her	Missed schooling (A) Ill health stopped family outings (A) Acute illness reinforces her disability (A)
Danger to self	Is able (with her mother's help) to manoeuvre herself in and out of bed and in and out of shower feels weak and unable to perform normal hygiene or mobility roles	Further breakdown of skin (P) Chest infection (P) Injury to herself and mother (P)

A, Actual problem; P, potential problem.

teenager, Tracy's wound care is similar to adult wound care with the same principles guiding the treatment.

Although Tracy has a whole host of medical problems, she also is an adolescent who has a right to be considered in all aspects of care.[3]

Orem's model can assist the nurse in her assessment to instigate the development of family-centred care. The nurse should be seen as the central 'facilitator' of care, not the main caregiver, and should be prepared to let go of tasks that may be seen traditionally as belonging to the nurse.

The first stage of the assessment establishes whether there is a deficit in Tracy's self-care abilities. Remember that we are also assessing Tracy's mother as the main caregiver.

Orem's model uses six universal self-care needs to make the assessment (Table 5.3). Having identified Tracy's problems, the nurse must decide why there is a self-care deficit. Is it due to a lack of knowledge, skills or motivation, or a limited range of behaviour? Tracy and her family were living a normal life before this period of hospitalization and they may need to learn new skills or new behaviour in order to resume that normalcy. By recognizing the cause of the problem, the district nurse can plan with Tracy and her mother a new course of action that is suited to all concerned.

The amount of intervention the nurse gives at this stage is crucial to the re-establishment of self-caring abilities.

Nursing intervention will be wholly compensatory, partly compensatory or educative/supportive (Table 5.4).

Practice Points

- In this case the district nurse's role has been mainly educative and partially compensatory. Even the wound care can be increasingly transferred to the mother.
- However, care must be taken that this role is willingly taken on. Often an acute episode like this triggers a breakdown in the family as the care unit.
- The nurse must assess the environment carefully and look for indications of strain and stress.

Road Traffic Accidents

Road traffic accidents are a common cause of traumatic wounds in teenagers and the associated problems are illustrated in Case Study 5.3.

EPIDEMIOLOGY

In the UK pedal cyclists killed on the roads in 2017 was slightly lower than in 2016, the 101 fatalities is very similar to the level seen since 2008.[16] Others experienced serious injuries. Head injuries are more common in young males than females at a ratio of 3:1, mostly affecting the 16–35-year age group. The incidence of death from head injury in the UK is low, with as few as 0.2% of all patients attending emergency departments with a head injury dying as a result of this injury.[17] Though many of these injuries are preventable. The use of crash helmets for motorcyclists and safety belts in cars has resulted in less serious injuries. A common factor that contributes to head injuries is overconsumption of alcohol.[18]

MANAGEMENT

Many patients seen in accident and emergency departments are fit, young individuals. Irrespective of the wound size, accurate assessment, diagnosis and thorough wound toilet must be achieved to ensure that any deficit in wound healing is identified and the appropriate treatment given.

Case Study 5.3

Road Traffic Accident

Darren Adams had been employed as a motorbike courier for the previous 6 months. Although he left school with three A Levels, he was unable to find employment for 12 months. Despite the job being unsuited to his capabilities, he was pleased to have some form of income until the right job came along.

Darren has always liked drinking with his friends but has usually been sensible enough to walk or take a taxi home. Last Friday, however, it was raining heavily and he did not have any money left for a taxi so he decided to ride his bike home. The roads were slippery and at a junction Darren pulled out in front of a car. The car braked but skidded into the bike, knocking Darren into the air some 2 metres before he landed on the bonnet of the car.

Darren was rushed to the local accident and emergency department. He was conscious, having sustained a fractured femur and severe lacerations to his face and arm. Following admission, Darren was informed that the police wished to interview him, at which point he became abusive and tried to throw himself off the trolley.

Before assessment of the traumatic wound is made, the patient's condition must be stabilized. Standard assessments of airway, breathing and circulation are made to ensure that all life-threatening conditions are identified. Any external bleeding is controlled with direct pressure on the wound. A thorough history of how the accident happened is then recorded, although this is difficult where a patient is unconsciousness and there are no witnesses. Other factors that are taken into account are:

- exact mechanism of injury
- amount of force
- foreign bodies in wound
- tendon or nerve damage
- time and place of accident.

It is important to establish whether the patient has any medical history of diabetes mellitus or epilepsy, is allergic to or is taking any particular medication.

Wound Assessment and Cleansing

All traumatic wounds will be contaminated by the time the patient arrives at the accident and emergency

TABLE 5.4   Nursing Interventions for Tracy (Case Study 5.2)

Self-Care Deficit	Goal	Interventions
Fluid Balance		
Needs extra fluids (lack of skill and motivation)	Tracy to be encouraged to drink as much as she can tolerate, aiming to reach 2 L daily	Supply of Tracy's favourite drinks to be available at bedside in vacuum flasks or large juice containers. 'Bendy' straws or sealed containers will aid drinking when lying in bed
Further urinary tract infection Renal failure (lack of knowledge)		Explore Tracy's and her mother's level of knowledge regarding the importance of keeping kidneys flushed with fluids. Use simple explanations without frightening them
Nutrition		
Weight loss (limited range of behaviour)	To regain previous weight	Increase energy content of diet to enhance weight gain, but avoid protein overload of kidneys. Contact community dietician to plan specific diet with family. Discuss with Tracy and her mother the effects of catabolism on wound healing
Catabolic state	To reduce the effects of catabolism and promote wound healing	
Poor diet (lack of knowledge)	To promote a healthier diet for future eating	Plan a diet with the family which will take into account finances, availability of foodstuffs and likes and dislikes
Elimination		
Cannot manage urostomy bag (limited range of behaviour)	Eliminate leakage	Reassess urostomy bag size and stoma. Refer to stoma-therapist for new appliance
Diarrhoea due to antibiotic (lack of knowledge)	Prevent diarrhoea	Explain importance of taking antibiotics at correct times. Advise Tracy to report any change in bowel motion
Increase of interface friction (lack of knowledge)	Reduce interface friction	Reinforce importance of skin cleansing following urine spillage
Activity and Rest		
Inadequate exercise (lack of motivation and limited behaviour) Muscle wasting (limited behaviour)	To resume 'normal' physical activity level	Resume daily routine of passive exercises of legs while in bed. Sit in chair for increasing periods each day, resuming arm lifts every half-hour. Discuss possibility of community physiotherapy weekly to keep motivation level high
Non-healing pressure ulcers (lack of knowledge)	To heal pressure ulcers	Reassess Tracy using identified risk assessment tool and review whether pressure-relieving equipment (bed and chair) meets her needs. Document wound position, size and tissue characteristics. Trace and/or photograph. Debride wound, using dressing material that will (i) keep wound occluded and prevent infection, (ii) minimize dressing changes, (iii) be possible for the mother to change if necessary, and (iv) provide comfort for Tracy
Further skin breakdown (lack of knowledge)	To prevent further ulcer development	Discuss with Tracy and her mother the reasons for initial ulcer development and indicators for prevention of future breakdown
Socializing		
Depressed owing to enforced hospitalization (lack of knowledge)	To introduce positive outlook on life	Encourage Tracy and her mother to reflect on the reasons why she went into hospital. Highlight the benefits of being home. Allow Tracy to work through her feelings, giving her time to talk

department[19] so an aseptic technique is not necessary until removal of gross contaminants is achieved.[20] The following is recommended practice:

- Foreign material should be removed by washing (irrigation; see Chapter 3), brushing or with forceps.
- Before further investigation is attempted the wound must be anaesthetized with plain lignocaine.
- All deeply embedded foreign bodies are removed and the damage examined in relation to underlying nerves and tendons.[18]
- Debridement of traumatized and devitalized tissue must be carried out, remembering that wound toilet should be directly proportional to the extent of contamination.[20]

Investigation

Radiographic investigation of traumatized limbs and suspected injury sites are required for an accurate diagnosis.

Antibiotics

Antibiotics are indicated for:

- infected wounds with systemic issues
- human or animal bites
- diabetic or immunocompromised patients.

Tetanus Prophylaxis

Tetanus prophylaxis may be considered for wounds more than 6 hours old that display:

- large amounts of devitalized tissue
- deep puncture-type injury such as a stab wound
- contact with soil or manure (e.g., in farm workers)
- evidence of infection
- severe burns
- human or animal bites.[18]

Nursing Model for Darren

Darren has sustained major injuries and requires a great deal of immediate treatment. Unfortunately for him, his arrival in the accident and emergency department has commenced with a confrontational event that is not conducive to developing a relationship with the nursing staff.

The nurse needs to calm Darren before treatment can begin and an assessment of his needs undertaken. The nurse should also consider the psychological consequences of labelling Darren as a drunken driver.

Darren has experienced a sudden change in circumstances from being a fit, healthy, intelligent young man. He is now immobile, facing criminal charges and potentially labelled as 'stupid' with no regard for the lives of others. He will need to adapt to ill health. Roy's adaptation model[21] may be used to assess and outline a plan of care (Table 5.5).

Practice Points

Before Darren can have an assessment of his traumatic injuries, the staff need to calm him as he is in grave danger of adding to his injuries.

Look at the assessment of his psychosocial status and identify the major problems:

- violent behaviour due to *shock, fear* and effects of *alcohol*
- placed in hospital surroundings which are *new* to him
- does not have any *family or friends* to provide *support*.

How can these problems be resolved?

Because of the way in which the traumatic injuries are incurred, patients are suddenly plunged into what may seem a hostile environment in the accident and emergency unit. This is compounded in Darren's case in that the police are also there waiting to see him.

Darren's wounds are debrided, irrigated and sutured. Antibiotic cover and frequent wound observation are instituted for the prevention and early detection of wound infection. In the long term the extent of Darren's scarring could have a lasting effect on his psychological state. Facial wounds often require the skills of a plastic surgeon using careful suturing techniques.

Most accident and emergency departments operate a triage system, enabling staff to prioritize patient care. Those requiring immediate emergency treatment are

TABLE 5.5   Assessment of Darren's Problems (Case Study 5.3) Using Roy's Adaptation Model

Life Area	Assessment Level 1 – Behaviour	Focal	Assessment level 2 – stimuli	
			Contextual	Residual
Self-concept	Abusive violent behaviour	Confrontation with A&E staff.	Staff not experienced in handling patient.	Social stigma of drunk driver.
	Fear of surroundings	Still in shock	A&E department	Never previously hospitalized
Role/function	Fears loss of job. Fears police conviction	Major traumatic injury. Knows he should not have driven	Extent of injury not assessed	No previous involve-ment with law
Interdependency	Dependent on staff, lack of self-control	Helpless owing to injuries and alcohol	Sudden change from being well to being seriously ill	Not 'normal' level of behaviour
Physiological	Multiple lacerations to face and arms	Contaminated wounds	Wounds embedded with grit and dirt from road	
	Pain	Compound fracture of femur	Further damage to underlying tissue	Length of time before arrival in A&E
	Contamination from road	Infection in wound		
	Hyperventilation	Fear and shock	Pain in leg	
	Feeling nauseated	Pain in leg. Shock	Effects of alcohol	

attended to first, while less urgent cases are dealt with later. In this case it might have been advisable to assess Darren's injuries and gain his confidence before the police were mentioned.

The priority of management is to ensure there are no life-threatening problems by using the 'ABC' protocol (airway, breathing and circulation), checking that there are no major bleeding points at the site of fracture and assessing previous blood loss. Vital signs are monitored for signs of shock, and the patient is calmed with the following:

- Reassurance: talk slowly, in a quiet area away from the hustle and bustle of the department. Enlist his trust – the nurse is there to help him.
- Pain relief: give appropriate analgesia if vital signs are satisfactory. Local analgesia may also be required before wound toilet is commenced at site of fracture.

- Explanation: explain the necessity to assess his injuries as quickly as possible and that this will require his cooperation. Ask him if he would like his family contacted.

Accident and emergency department staff are trained to provide reassurance and gain the patient's trust quickly, while simultaneously performing resuscitation techniques.

Look at the physiological areas of assessment. The important points here are:

- wound cleansing and wound toilet
- thorough examination of lacerations and extent of injuries
- antibiotic and tetanus cover
- accurate documentation of both events of accident and nature of injury.

Devise the care plan, taking these points into account. Look at the assessment in Table 5.5 if you need help.

Summary

Injury to teenagers can be both physiologically and psychologically traumatic. The nurse has an important role to play in providing skilled management of the wound and gaining the patient's trust. The bond that can develop between nurse and teenager can be rewarding and enhance the level of care given.

The important issues to remember when dealing with the cases outlined can be summarized as follows:

- Gain the trust of the teenager before commencement of any treatment.
- Ensure that adequate pain relief is always given.
- Consider the effects that immobility or scarring may have on them for the rest of their lives.
- Be aware that teenagers can easily be emotionally crushed; always communicate in a clear and understanding way.
- Documentation, as always, is of utmost importance. Claims may be made many years on from the actual date of the accident or injury.
- Be aware that inadequate management may result in inadequate wound healing.

FURTHER READING

Gowar JP, Lawrence JC. The incidence, cause and treatment of minor burns. *J Wound Care*. 1995;4(2):71–74

Wardrope J, Smith J. *The Management of Wounds and Burns*. Oxford: Oxford University Press; 1993.

Wright B. *Caring in Crisis: A Handbook of Intervention Skills*. 2nd ed. Edinburgh: Churchill Livingstone; 1993.

REFERENCES

1. Hazinski MF. *Manual of Pediatric Critical Care*. St Louis, MO: Mosby; 1999.
2. Wheal A. Adolescents. In: *Adolescence: Positive Approaches for Working with Young People*. Lyme Regis, UK: Russell House Publishing; 1999.
3. Taylor J, Muller D, Wattley L, Harris P. The adolescent in hospital. In: *Nursing Children*. London: Stanley Thornes; 1999.
4. Eurostat, Being young in Europe today - health, 2018. available under: https://ec.europa.eu/eurostat/statistics-explained/index.php/Being_young_in_Europe_today_-_health#Causes_of_death.
5. Helath and Safety Executive (HSE) Workplace fatal injuries in Great Britain, 2019 available under: https://www.hse.gov.uk/statistics/pdf/fatalinjuries.pdf.
6. Helath and Safety Executive (HSE) Reporting accidents and incidents at work 2013. available under: https://www.hse.gov.uk/pubns/indg453.pdf.
7. Petch N, Cason CG. Examining first aid received by burn and scald patients. *J Wound Care*. 1993;2(2):102–105.
8. Mertens DM, Jenkins ME, Warden GD. Outpatient burns management. *Nurs Clin North Am*. 1997;32(2):343–364.
9. Dowsett C. The assessment and management of burns. *Br J Community Nurs*. 2002;7(5):230–239.
10. McCormack A, La Hei ER, Martin HC. First-aid management of minor burns in children: a prospective study of children presenting to the Children's Hospital at Westmead, Sydney. *Med J Aust*. 2003;178(1):31–33.
11. Roper N, Logan WW, Tierney AJ. *The Elements of Nursing*. 4th ed. Edinburgh: Churchill Livingstone; 1996.
12. Spina Bifida Association 2020. available under: https://www.spinabifidaassociation.org/.
13. Pieper B. Mechanical forces: pressure, shear, and friction. In: Bryant RA, ed. *Acute and Chronic Wounds: Nursing Management*. St Louis, MO: Mosby; 2000.
14. National Pressure Ulcer Advisory Panel. European Pressure Ulcer Advisory Panel and Pan Pacific Pressure Injury Alliance. In: Haesler E, ed. *Prevention and Treatment of Pressure Ulcers: Quick Reference Guide*. Osborne Park, Australia: Cambridge Media; 2014. Available at: http://www.epuap.org/pu-guidelines/.
15. Department of Transport. Reported road casualties in Great Britain: 2017 annual report, 2018. Available under: https://assets.publishing.service.gov.uk/government/uploads/system/uploads/attachment_data/file/744077/reported-road-casualties-annual-report-2017.pdf.
16. Allan D. The nervous system. In: Alexander MR, Fawcett JN, Runciman PJ, eds. *Nursing Practice*. Edinburgh: Churchill Livingstone; 1999.
17. NICE guidance: Head injury: assessment and early management, updated version 2019. CG 176 available under: https://www.nice.org.uk/guidance/cg176/chapter/Introduction.
18. Bale S, Leaper D. Acute wounds. In: Bale S, Harding K, Leaper D, eds. *An Introduction to Wounds*. London: Emap Healthcare Ltd; 2000.
19. Dealey C. The management of patients with chronic wounds. In: *The Care of Wounds*. Oxford: Blackwell Science; 1999.
20. Ayello EA, Baranoski S, Kerstein MD, Cuddigan J. Wound debridement. In: Baranoski S, Ayello EA, eds. *Wound Care Essentials: Practice Principles*. Springhouse, PA: Lippincott, Williams and Wilkins; 2004.
21. Roy C, Andrews H. *The Roy Adaptation Model*. 2nd ed. Stamford, CT: Appleton and Lange; 1999.

MCQS

1 *What is the most common cause of wounds in adolescent patients?*
   a. Trauma/accident
   b. Chronic disease
   c. Spinal cord injury
   d. Tumour/cancer-related issues

2 *Burns are an major cause trauma-based wounds in teenagers. Which of the following would be most effective in helping prevent such injuries?*
   a. Smoking prevention campaigns targeted at teens
   b. Prevention strategies aimed at teenage girls because these injuries most affect girls in this age group
   c. Prevention strategies targeting those in early childhood so that they grow into teenagers who are aware of the risks
   d. Prevention strategies aimed at teenage boys, especially with regard to accidental and unsafe handling of fire, fireworks and chemicals

3 *What is the main aim of the organization Changing Faces?*
   a. To increase preventive interventions in community areas
   b. To highlight the issue of stigmatization by visible wounds, scars and skin deformities and support peoples' self-confidence
   c. To provide information to schools and community services about burns treatments
   d. To support research in tissue biology

Chapter 6

Wound Care in the Young Adult

Anna-Barbara Schlüer

Highlights

As you read through this chapter concentrate on the following:

- The effects emergency surgery may have on postoperative wound management
- Factors that should be considered in preoperative management that enhance postoperative care
- The effect a wound can have on the patient's normal living pattern
- The range of dressings available that patients can manage themselves
- The importance of including the patient in planning care

Key Issues

This chapter examines the type of wound management required by the young adult.

Clinical Case Studies

Aetiology and management of:

- A 22-year-old man requiring emergency excision of a pilonidal sinus
- A woman with postoperative wound problems after an emergency caesarean section
- A 36-year-old man with a traumatic injury following an accident that requires preparation for plastic surgery
- A woman with a self-inflicted leg wound

Nursing Models

Examples of their application to practice are taken from:

- Orem's model
- Roy's adaptation model
- Riehl-Sisca's interaction model

Introduction

Young adulthood is a stage in the life cycle where the individual feels immune to disease and ill health. The young value their youthfulness and vigour and generally thrive on fitness. For the young, the image of a sick individual may be one of a helpless, older person being the passive recipient of both medical and nursing care. Young adults, if needing healthcare, are likely to challenge this dynamic. They feel confident, empowered and expect to become involved in making decisions about their care and management. Patients and health professionals are encouraged to work together in partnership,[1,2] so that patients have the opportunity to make informed choices about their care. Nurses should ensure that, as with all patients, young adults are engaged in making decisions about their wound care.

Preparing for Planned Surgery

Surgical procedures may be offered to many young people with a variety of health problems. For many problems that are not life threatening, the decision to accept or refuse surgery rests solely with the individual. Examples of these problems include lipomas and ingrowing toenails; the patient will decide how troublesome it is. Other health problems such as inguinal hernia, ovarian cyst and pilonidal sinus may lead to further complications and are best treated with surgical intervention. Individuals vary greatly in their response to the prospect of surgery: some regard it in a matter-of-fact way, others with great fear and trepidation. Experience in childhood or the experiences of family members or friends is often an influencing factor – it may generate confidence and reassurance or perhaps fear and mistrust.

Great advances have been made in surgical procedures. The use of the laparoscope for 'keyhole' surgery has enabled knee surgery and abdominal surgery to be carried out through very small incisions. Where appropriate, such operations can take place in day surgery units where the patient does not stay overnight. From a cost-saving point of view, there is an increasing trend for young, fit individuals to be offered day surgery. From the patient's point of view, the advantages include a short stay in hospital, reduced pain and immobility, and an earlier return to normal activities.

Patients requiring more extensive surgery will need to be admitted to a surgical ward. Preoperatively the nurse has an important role to play in helping to prepare the patient for surgery. As well as the physical assessment, the nurse can provide information and emotional support on admission. It is well documented that with information and support given to reduce stress and anxiety, the patient has a much better postoperative outcome.[3] It is also important to bear in mind that the perspective of a surgeon is not the same as that of the patient. The surgeon is often focused on the technicalities of performing the best surgery possible and on a good outcome. Aspects such as postoperative pain, postoperative immobility, patients' anxieties and their long-term care, including skin and scar care, is often not the primary focus of the surgeon.

Interruption of daily activities may be perceived as problematic for the young individual. With planning, education need not be disrupted and it is usual for young patients to be offered a date for surgery to coincide with university and college holidays. Concern may be focused around the length of time that a favourite sport may not be played or when they may be able to socialize.

Linked to this may be concerns about altered body image. The young value their youth, health, beauty and vigour[4] and any disfigurement, however minor, may have a disproportionately negative effect. By providing the necessary support, it is in this area that nursing can significantly improve the experience and outcome for young adults undergoing straightforward surgical procedures.

There are on the horizon some less invasive and more advanced technology-based interventions that will benefit young adults with wounds and scarring issues. For example, the use of CO_2 lasers looks set to have an immense

---

Case Study 6.1

Emergency Excision of Pilonidal Sinus

Colin Sharples is a 22-year-old law student just entering his final year of studies. A fit, healthy young man who has always been involved in many sporting activities, he has never had any experience of illness or hospitalization.

During the past 6 months he has had a feeling of discomfort in his natal cleft which appears to come and go and is often associated with feeling generally unwell. Last week the discomfort became an acute, stabbing pain which prevented him from sitting down. He went to the college doctor who diagnosed his condition as pilonidal disease and gave him a course of antibiotics. Unfortunately Colin took his antibiotics for only 2 days as he felt better and did not really like taking tablets. Within a week he was admitted to hospital for an emergency wide excision of a pilonidal abscess.

Following surgery the wound was left to heal by secondary intention and measured 10 cm in length by 3 cm breadth and 4 cm depth. Colin was extremely anxious postoperatively and, although in pain, was reluctant to stay in hospital as he wanted to resume his studies. Furthermore, Colin was embarrassed about the wound and its location. Once back at home this impacted on his post-intervention wound care, as he avoided help from a community nurse and the location of the wound meant it was difficult for Colin to care for the wound himself.

---

impact on the treatment of keloids and hypertrophic scarring. The use of advanced wound treatment will in some circumstances replace surgical intervention.

Coping with Emergency Surgery

The onset of an acute illness or trauma can result in the need for emergency surgery. An example is given in Case Study 6.1. Preparation of the young person as described above may not be possible and often only brief, essential information can be given in the immediate preoperative period. In the postoperative period patients are likely to have many questions, which could need answering several times as the patient recovers from both the anaesthesia and surgery.

AETIOLOGY

Pilonidal sinus disease commonly affects young adults, arising at some time after puberty, and is rarely found after the age of 40 years. Men are affected by pilonidal

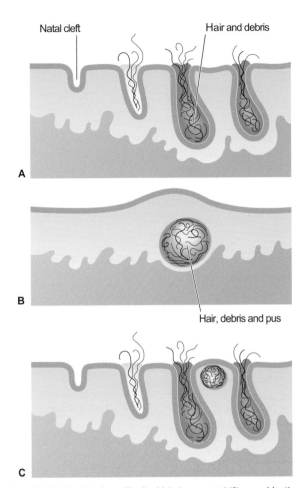

Fig. 6.1 (A) Pilonidal sinus; (B) pilonidal abscess; and (C) a combination of pilonidal sinus with pilonidal abscess.

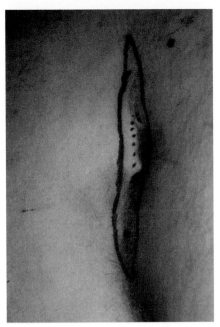

Fig. 6.2 Pilonidal sinus disease prior to surgery. Marked on the patient's skin is the area to be excised, together with the sites of individual sinuses.

sinus disease around ten times more than women and it is associated with having a sedentary occupation, a family history, obesity and local irritation or trauma prior to onset of symptoms.[5] Around 75% of those undergoing surgery are males and 25% are females [6] Pilonidal sinus disease causes a great deal of suffering, inconvenience, loss of time from work and loss of income, as patients can have problems for up to 3 years. Patients generally present with recurrent pain and purulent discharge.[7] The recurrence rate following excision can be as high as 50%[8] and with reconstructive skin flaps as low as 5%.[9]

There are several theories as to why pilonidal sinus disease occurs, the most likely being that it is an acquired disease (Fig. 6.1). With the onset of puberty, sex hormones begin to act on pilosebaceous glands

in the natal cleft. With this a hair follicle becomes distended with keratin and subsequently infected, so resulting in a folliculitis and an abscess that extends down into subcutaneous fat.[5] In 93%, the direction of the abscess and secondary tracts follows the orientation of the inflamed hair follicles. The abscess is likely to drain out onto the skin through the tract.[10] Hairs are drilled or sucked into the abscess cavity through friction with movement of the buttocks. This process encourages loose debris and other body hair to enter and accumulate in the sinus (Fig. 6.2). Most commonly *Staphylococcus aureus* and *Bacteroides* are the pathogens causing the infection. Patients may be asymptomatic for some time before presenting with local discomfort and/or discharge. However, about 50% of patients present with an acute pilonidal abscess.

MANAGEMENT

There are a number of surgical techniques available, although no one procedure has been demonstrated to be better than another overall. It is generally agreed that the most effective emergency management of a pilonidal abscess is simple incision and drainage.[5] However, the treatment of chronic and recurrent pilonidal disease is more difficult and the options include excision with primary closure or healing by secondary intention, Lord's procedure, phenol injections and skin flaps.[11–13]

Several treatments may be offered to patients:

- Curettage for small, non-infected sinuses: it may be possible to remove the hairs with a pair of forceps and brushing out tracts. Lord's procedure is one such treatment that is reported to be associated with 80–90% healing.[7]
- Excision and primary closure: here the sinuses are excised and the wound edges brought together and sutured. This procedure can result in 70% healing at 2 weeks, although 20% of patients develop a wound infection.[9,12–14]
- Wide excision and laying open of the sinuses together with the skin: all tissues are excised down to the sacrum.[5] The patient requires frequent dressing changes and a great deal of support. This procedure is associated with 70–90% healing at 70 days and a recurrence rate of 5–15%.[7]

As Colin's disease was widespread, the wide excision technique was used, leaving a large cavity wound (Figs 6.3–6.6).

Local Wound Management

This large cavity will take about 6–8 weeks to heal by secondary intention. With care Colin could return to fairly normal activities quickly and could take responsibility for his own wound hygiene. Some of the dressing materials that could be used include the following:

- Days 0–2: alginate materials, especially those containing sodium, are useful haemostatic agents. The dressing can be packed into the wound immediately following surgery, in the operating theatre, to achieve haemostasis. After 48 hours this alginate packing can be washed out of the cavity using warm saline.
- Day 2 onwards through the proliferative phase: alginate and hydrofibre materials can be used but this treatment needs a nurse to change the dressings. Other useful materials include cavity foam dressings and occasionally a hydrogel. Foam dressings, especially disposable and those formed *in situ*, can be managed by patients on a daily basis and so

facilitate early return to normal activity. The main function of a cavity dressing for a pilonidal sinus excision is to keep the wound edges apart as healing takes place, so preventing superficial bridges and the possibility of a dead space in the depths of the wound. Wound hygiene is of particular importance, as is regular inspection and assessment of the granulation tissue to detect the early signs of clinical infection.[5] Here, the signs of clinical infection include the presence of flimsy, friable, discoloured granulation tissue; bleeding; superficial bridging; pain; and increased exudate production.[15] In the long term, after the acute wound has healed, a treatment with intense pulsed light (IPL) laser is suggested for prevention of relapse.

Nursing Model for Colin

Colin is a normal, fit, healthy young adult who does not really want to be in hospital or have his normal routine altered. The following are likely to be some of his concerns:

- disruption of his studies
- disruption of his sporting activities
- disruption of sexual activity
- embarrassment at exposing buttocks to nurses
- lack of privacy in hospital
- likelihood of recurrence of disease
- length of time in hospital
- stigmatization
- worry about being dependent on long-term care.

Colin's major worries are not directly concerned with wound management. In a fit, healthy young man this open granulating wound should heal easily and without complication.

Practice Points

You should have identified Colin's self-care deficit from the list of main concerns. The management that Colin needs, therefore, should be along the following lines:

- Following an initial 3–4 days in hospital Colin can be discharged with arrangements made with the community nurse or university campus nurse to continue care.
- Initially the wound could be packed with alginates to achieve haemostasis; then, in the following few days, a cavity foam dressing could be introduced. Colin could change these dressings himself, following daily showering.

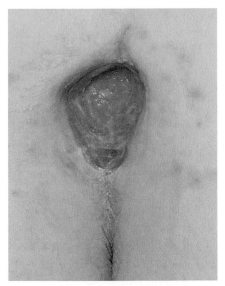

Fig. 6.3 Wide excision of pilonidal sinus at week 2.

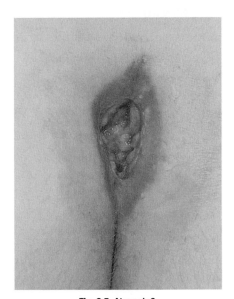

Fig. 6.5 At week 6.

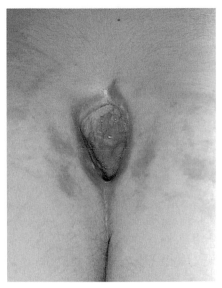

Fig. 6.4 At week 4,

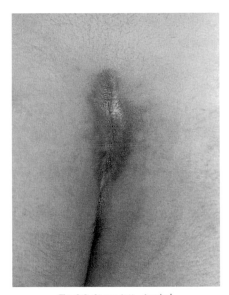

Fig. 6.6 At week 8 – healed.

He needs to understand that strenuous exercise must be avoided for up to 12 weeks.
- Colin requires a flexible approach to his care, the need to feel in control and the assurance that he has professional advice when needed.

- Orem's model would fulfil these needs, with an early discharge into the community under the care of the university campus nurse and specialist outpatient visits at frequent intervals.

Caesarean Section

Case Study 6.2 discusses the problems arising from wound breakdown after an apparently straightforward caesarean section.

AETIOLOGY

Normal spontaneous vaginal delivery remains constant at around 66% of all births in the UK.[16] Caesarean section is the operation by which a potentially viable fetus is delivered through an incision in the abdominal wall and uterus. It is indicated for fetal compromise, failure to progress in labour (dystocia), previous caesarean section and breech presentation.[16] However, the gradual increase in the incidence of caesarean sections to 21% globally in 2015 is of concern.[17] Guidelines recommend that when indicated, the benefits, risks and the evidence base for different interventions of caesarean section should be discussed with the woman and also where women request a caesarean section without good clinical reason. In order to decrease morbidity from caesarean section, regional anaesthesia should be used in conjunction with antibiotic prophylaxis, antacids and antiemetics.[17]

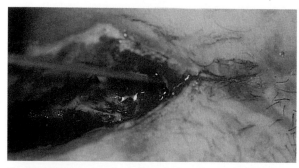

Fig. 6.7 Kate Hemmings' wound, showing a probe inserted into the undermining area.

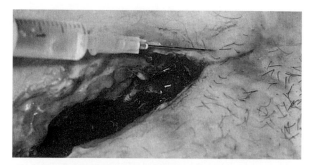

Fig. 6.8 Local anaesthetic being injected into the area to be incised.

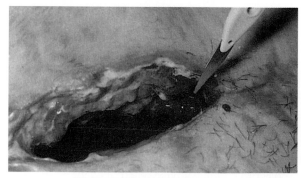

Fig. 6.9 Incising the undermined area.

Case Study 6.2

Caesarean Section

Mrs Kate Hemmings, a 34-year-old, gave birth to her third child by emergency caesarean section. Kate had a caesarean delivery with her first child but delivered her second child normally and had wanted to try and deliver this baby normally also. Following 7 days in hospital, Kate and baby Julia were discharged home into the care of the community staff.

Her sutures were removed at 10 days with the wound apparently having healed without any complications. She felt well in herself, albeit a little tired, but felt this was to be expected with a small baby and two other toddlers to cope with.

By the 12th day she noticed a small red spot in the middle of the scar line which, following a bath, began to ooze fluid. Alarmed at this, she called the district nurse who placed a dressing pad on the area.

Over the following week the oozing continued and an opening became visible which measured 2 cm in width when probed. The surrounding wound area was hard and red and Kate was feeling generally unwell. The district nurse probed the wound and found it undermined 1 cm either side of the scar line (Fig. 6.7). The nurse called the GP who admitted Kate to the gynaecology ward at the local hospital. The wound was opened up 1.5 cm either side of the gaping edge to make a small cavity to facilitate drainage of exudate (Figs 6.8–6.10). The wound was packed with an alginate dressing and on Kate's insistence, she was discharged home 48 hours later.

The most common surgical technique employed is the lower segment caesarean section (Fig. 6.11). A transverse abdominal incision 3 cm above the symphysis pubis is the technique of choice as this is associated with shorter operating times, reduced bleeding, reduced postoperative morbidity and pain, and an improved cosmetic effect.[17] Postoperative infection is also reduced because the lower segment is outside the peritoneal cavity.

MANAGEMENT

Normally wound management would entail removal of sutures at between 10 and 14 days. Here, however, as with

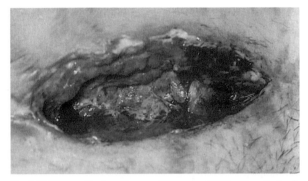

Fig. 6.10 The resultant cavity wound is now a suitable shape for healing by secondary intention.

breakdown of surgical wounds, it is advisable to incise the wound to allow free drainage of exudate (see Chapter 3).

This type of wound can be managed using an alginate packing dressing gently inserted into the undermining wound. The function of the dressing in this situation is to maintain a channel through which infected exudate can drain and to allow the wound to heal from its depths. It is probably advisable to irrigate the cavity daily with water or saline prior to repacking. This will rinse out any fragments of alginate left in the wound and also flush away bacteria. Alternatively, a hydrogel could be introduced into the wound to act as packing. Again, daily irrigation would be beneficial. Due to pregnancy-related hormonal changes in the skin, postnatal wounds sometimes heal inconsistently and follow an unusual healing pathway. The overstretching of tissues in pregnancy also makes the skin, especially the dermis, more susceptible to inflammatory responses. The aetiology of these processes are not fully understood.

Nursing Model for Kate

It is obvious that Kate has a postoperative wound infection that requires immediate treatment. However, having had to leave her baby, two young children and husband at home, she insisted on returning home within 48 hours.

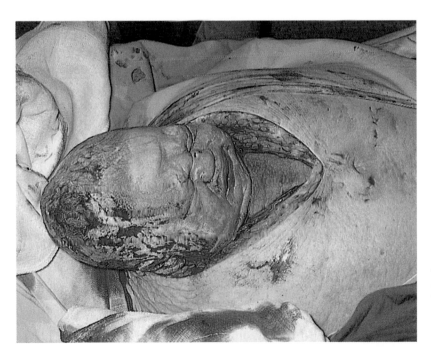

Fig. 6.11 The lower uterine segment has been excised transversely and the large fetal head, directly occipitoposterior, has been delivered by manual extraction. (Reproduced with kind permission from Beischer NA, Mackay EV. *Obstetrics and the Newborn: An Illustrated Textbook.* 2nd revised ed. London: Bailliere Tindall; 1986.)

TABLE 6.1 Assessment of Mrs Hemmings' Problems (Case Study 6.2) Using Orem's Model

Self-Care Need	Self-Care Ability	Self-Care Deficit
Nutrition	Little time to eat with three children (P) Little appetite owing to infection (A) Losing nutrients through breastfeeding (A)	Inadequate diet (A) Anaemia (P) Unable to breastfeed (P)
Activity and rest	Not sleeping because of new baby (P) Worried infection will be passed to baby (P)	Delay in wound healing due to lack of sleep (A) Unable to play with children and baby (P)
Socializing	Unable to go out with baby owing to wound infection (A)	Depression (P) No normal mother–baby activities (A)
Normalcy	Needs to wait in for nurse to do dressings	Feels restricted Cannot get into routine with other children and baby

A, Actual problem; P, potential problem.

It is important to provide her with a flexible form of management that allows her to cope at home. She needs to feel in control of her own care but obviously requires support, both emotionally and physically, from family and health professions.

Before choosing a model of care, ask yourself the following questions:

- Will Kate be able, or want, to change the dressing herself?
- How will the presence of the wound infection affect the young baby?
- What were the possible reasons for her developing this infection?
- Why is it better that Kate stays at home during her recovery?

Orem's model[18] addresses Kate's problems, as she will probably be motivated to achieve self-care (Table 6.1).

Practice Point

You must plan the management in such a way that Kate can resume her way of life as quickly as possible.

Traumatic Injury

The nature of traumatic injury results in a shocked and seriously ill patient who needs emergency surgery followed by preparation for planned plastic surgery, as in the example in Case Study 6.3.

AETIOLOGY

Among 26–45 year olds, for the year 2016, around 332 people died each year in the United States of America

Case Study 6.3

Emergency and Planned Surgery

Mr Jeremy Watkins is a married man of 36 years of age with three children aged 10, 7 and 3. Most of his adult life he has enjoyed water sports, although since the children arrived he has only been able to pursue this interest a few times a year.

He was with two friends taking a 3-day water sports holiday in Wales and canoeing down a river when his canoe overturned and he was crushed against sharp rocks. His friends and the instructor rushed to his assistance to find him shocked, bleeding heavily from his right thigh and on the verge of unconsciousness. The instructor and his friends dragged him out of the water and off the rocks, applied pressure to the large gash and summoned help. On admission to hospital, Jeremy was found to have lost some muscle, subcutaneous fat and skin from his thigh, as well as a significant amount of blood. He was transfused and taken to theatre where an orthopaedic surgeon and a plastic surgeon assessed the damage to his leg. A negative-pressure wound therapy (NPWT) was applied. By the time Jeremy returned from the recovery room, his wife had travelled 60 miles to be with him, leaving their children with friends.

(USA) from drowning in boating-related incidents.[19] In 2010 the American Canoe Association reported that approximately 90% of all canoeing-related fatality victims were not wearing a life jacket at the time of the accident and that occupant movement and weight shift within a canoe played a major role in roughly 50% of all canoeing accidents.

MANAGEMENT

Following surgical excision of the devitalized skin, muscle and subcutaneous tissues, the wound was packed for 48–72 hours to achieve haemostasis; haemostatic alginate dressings are useful for this purpose. As the wound was extensive, copious amounts of wound exudate were produced. A comfortable, soft, absorbent dressing that could be used throughout most of the healing phase is a hydrophilic foam, which was packed into the wound. Without the loss of muscle and subcutaneous tissue, Jeremy would have been able to achieve complete healing using dressings and could have been discharged from hospital a few days postoperatively. However, due to the extensive loss of tissue, Jeremy was referred to the plastic surgeon for reconstructive plastic surgery. In order to control the excessive exudate, prepare the wound bed and ensure that no infection would jeopardize this surgery, it was decided to use topical negative-pressure wound therapy (NPWT). The NPWT system was obtained under the trust's equipment provision contract and applied to the wound for 12 days. Following this treatment the wound bed was clean, healthy and granulating and Jeremy was transferred to his local hospital which had a plastic surgery unit attached to it.

In the immediate postoperative period, movement was difficult and painful but as time passed this dramatically improved. Provision of adequate, regular analgesia and gentle repositioning helped keep Jeremy as comfortable as possible.

Nursing Model for Jeremy

Look back at Jeremy's case. You will notice that the following features stand out about this patient:

- He has endured *shock* and distress due to the unexpected nature of his accident.
- He has *dependent children.*
- He has undergone emergency surgery and has *waited* almost 2 weeks for this operation.
- He *needs/wants* to go *home.*
- He has *limited* range of *movement.*

Jeremy needs to go home but will require much support from the community nurses. He is a strong, determined man and is used to being completely independent. Problems could develop if he chooses not to follow the community nurse's advice on wound care. The following are essential aspects of Jeremy's ongoing nursing care:

Case Study 6.4

Self-Inflicted Injury

Justina Finlay presented to her GP with an area of necrotic tissue above the inside of her left ankle. On examination, the wound was found to be 4 cm in diameter with a surrounding area of inflamed tissue. The GP did not know Justina very well but took only a brief history and sent her to the practice nurse for a dressing.

Justina did not go into the practice nurse's treatment room that day but presented herself 3 days later in a somewhat anxious state. Charge Nurse Andrews, an experienced nurse who has worked both in general nursing and psychiatry, sat Justina down and, before looking at her wound, spent some time asking her about her medical and social history.

Justina is unemployed and lives in a small caravan with some friends on the outskirts of the town. She stated that she cut her ankle while chopping wood and had tried to dress it herself but that it had turned septic-looking and was now black.

Examination of the wound revealed widespread cellulitis and phlebitis surrounding an obviously infected, necrotic wound (Fig. 6.12). Charge Nurse Andrews attempted mechanical debridement of the wound but this was too painful and Justina became agitated and threatened to leave the surgery. The nurse measured Justina's temperature (which was 39.5°C) and blood pressure; while doing so she noticed needle marks covering the arm.

- The nurse learns the nature of the difficulty the patient is experiencing.
- The nurse and patient develop a mutual trust.
- The nurse can then identify the patient's problems.

Practice Point

Using the SOAP assessment framework (see Chapter 2), plan Jeremy's care.

Factitious Wounds

Factitious or self-inflicted wounds can pose enormous problems to healthcare staff, as shown in Case Study 6.4.

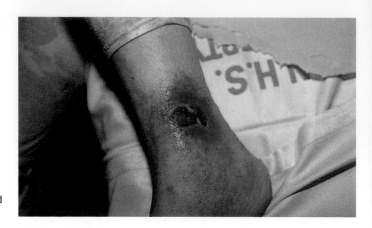

Fig. 6.12 Justina Finlay's ankle showing self-inflicted wound following assumed intravenous drug abuse.

AETIOLOGY

It is a common assumption by clinicians that achievement of wound healing is a shared goal or outcome of both the patient with the wound and the professionals caring for that patient.[20] However, for a small percentage of patients this is not the case. A minority of individuals may be responsible for either creating a wound or preventing an existing wound from healing.

More than 24,000 teenagers are admitted annually to hospital after deliberately harming themselves and around 1 in 10 self-harm.[21] Young people who self-harm are trying to communicate how they feel inside and are having difficulties in doing so, and they often need professional help to achieve this.[22] One study established the incidence of factitious wounds as being 0.5% of non-healing wounds attending a specialist wound clinic.[23] This study reported that although the mean age at which patients received treatment for their factitious wounds was 44 years, the mean age of onset of the wounds was much lower, at 34 years, with equal numbers of men and women presenting.

Young patients had a particular set of social circumstances thought to be associated with their psychiatric illness. All young people were single and still living at home with their parents. For this young group of patients the average age of onset of the non-healing wound was 20 years and these individuals demonstrated limited social maturity and found difficulties in forming personal relationships outside their family group. As this illness progresses the young individual becomes increasingly socially isolated and dependent on both family and healthcare professionals. Should the true nature of the non-healing wound be suspected and the patient confronted, denial is likely to be rapidly followed by the patient seeking referral to another healthcare professional.[22]

Although tempting, direct confrontation is not an effective approach for young individuals with factitious wounds. An alternative approach has been put forward[20] in which the nurse or doctor informs the patient that they know what might have caused the wound not to heal but also, at the same time, offers an alternative explanation. A new wound treatment is then prescribed and the patient is told that if this new treatment is not effective that self-inflicted injury will be confirmed. This approach is helpful by offering the patient the choice of either stopping interfering with the wound or accepting the opportunity to receive psychotherapy. It also avoids the patient transferring to another healthcare professional for the cycle to be repeated.

MANAGEMENT

The long-term outcome for these young patients is poor, with many wounds staying unhealed for some time.

This is undoubtedly a very difficult aspect of care to manage. Accurate documentation of the patient and wound assessment is crucial. The experienced nurse may identify a situation in which the appearance of the wound and the history the patient gives do not correspond. The first line of management should be to exclude physical causes for non-healing, which are often difficult to detect, and to obtain as much information as possible from previous medical and nursing notes.

TABLE 6.2   Identification of Justina's Problems (Case Study 6.4)

Psychological	Physical	Sociological
Denial of cause of wound (A) Barrier between nurse and patient (A) Requires help for wound but reluctant to seek it (A) Stigma associated with type of wound (A) Fear of drug problem being exposed (A)	Necrotic non-healing wound (A) Localized infection (A) Invasive infection and septicaemia (P) Loss of use of foot/limb (P) Infection with HIV/AIDS (A or P) Addiction to abusive substance (A)	Involved in drug-taking subculture (A) Not in long-term employment (A) Lives in squalid housing conditions (A)

A, Actual problem; P, potential problem.

Remember that the patient may have received treatment in other hospitals or other parts of the country. Systemic and local infections need to be promptly treated as serious illness could result from such infection.

Above all, the nurse's manner and approach to the young individual in these difficult circumstances need careful thought. It is important for the nurse not to judge the patient by their own standards and to appreciate the complex nature of factitious illness.

The use of dressings which require infrequent changes with the minimum of fuss take the focus away from the wound. Occlusive dressings, such as hydrocolloids, also prevent the transmission of bacteria from the environment to the wound bed and help prevent the patient interfering with the wound.

Nursing Model for Justina

Look back over this young woman's history. What do you suspect may be the cause of her wound?

The obvious conclusion would be that she is an injecting drug abuser and has used her leg veins for access. However, unless Justina is prepared to give Charge Nurse Andrews this information, how can it be proved?

The critical element of this case will be the nurse–patient interaction; so, Charge Nurse Andrews can use the Riehl interaction model.[24] The key information to be collected is the patient's 'definition' of the situation; therefore the nurse must attempt to enter into the patient's world in order to understand her viewpoint. Riehl underplays the physiological systems as the determinants of patients' problems, emphasizing the importance of psychosocial aspects.

In the first stage of the assessment it is necessary to ascertain whether Justina is adopting an appropriate role for her situation.

- Assessment (stage 1): Is Justina adopting an appropriate role for her present situation?
  - (No)
- Planning (stage 2): What are her problems related to?
  - Physical? (Yes)
  - Psychological? (Yes)
  - Sociological? (Yes).

It is necessary to identify the problems (Table 6.2) and negotiate person-centred goals (Table 6.3).

Practice Points

- Justina belongs to a subculture where drug taking is the norm and personal self-esteem is low.
- Charge Nurse Andrews attempts to build a relationship with Justina by involving her in her care and seeking her opinion.
- She realizes that Justina may not attend the surgery again, so attempts to teach her some kind of self-care but also liaises with the community nurses. Much of her care is a form of role play because she demonstrates to Justina that she is non-judgemental about her drug abuse but cares about her physical condition.
- She cannot cure the drug problem but she provides opportunities for Justina to seek help if desired.
- The wound may not heal, especially if Justina tries to gain access to a vein in the same site.
- The overall aim of management, therefore, is not necessarily wound healing but to gain the patient's trust so that her real problem (drug abuse) can be dealt with.

TABLE 6.3 Person-Centred Goals and Interventions Planned for Justina (Case Study 6.4)

Goal	Intervention
Psychological	
Enable patient to reveal her problem of drug abuse by forming a trusting relationship between nurse and patient	• Display a non-judgemental attitude to Justina when attending to the wound • Give ample opportunity for Justina to discuss her problems • Stress confidentiality of treatment and any patient details recorded • Ensure treatment time will be undisturbed by other members of the practice • Indicate that you are aware of her problem, but will only discuss it if she wishes • Allow Justina to see her records – do not hide them from her
To form a trusting relationship between nurse and patient	• Display a concerned attitude towards Justina's general physical and mental condition • Involve Justina in planning care for her wound and seek her opinion • Explain the nature of wound healing and the risk of possible infection • Ensure Justina knows whom to contact if the condition of the wound deteriorates • Encourage Justina to discuss her relationship with family and friends • Ensure that she is given correct information regarding the treatment plan
Physiological	
Removal of necrotic tissue to promote healing of wound	• Cover wound with a hydrocolloid dressing to promote autolysis and provide a protective barrier • Take a wound swab to confirm the type of organisms present in the wound • Teach Justina safe methods of cleaning her wound and reapplying the dressing (role play) • Liaise with community nurses to arrange home visits • Document size, site and appearance of wound on initial and subsequent visits
To prevent spread of infection systemically	• Explain the importance of keeping the wound clean • Ensure use of gloves when removing and reapplying dressings • Doctor to prescribe course of prophylactic antibiotics • Explain importance of taking antibiotic cover • Arrange a mutually convenient time for Justina to attend the surgery
Sociological	
To facilitate opportunities for Justina to improve her socio-economic status	• Provide information regarding helplines, drug counsellors, etc. • Ensure Justina has appropriate benefit entitlement

Summary

This chapter has reflected on four different examples of the range of wound care situations encountered by young adults.

Healing will mostly take place in this age group without too many physiological complications; however, psychological and sociological problems will require as much if not more attention to ensure the patient reaches a satisfactory outcome.

The models used here highlight the following important aspects of wound care in this group of patients:

• patient and nurse planning care together to meet the patient's needs

• the nurse aiming to understand the problems from the patient's perspective
• the effect the wound will have on the patient's normal living patterns
• the range of available dressings that the patient can manage alone
• the nurse remaining non-judgemental and using counselling skills to gain the patient's trust.

These are skills that are gained through clinical experience and reflective practice. Look for somebody in your clinical area who you feel possesses these skills and watch how they interact with their patients.

FURTHER READING

Dealey C. *The Care of Wounds*. Oxford: Blackwell Scientific; 1999.

Eagle M. The care of a patient after a caesarean section. *J Wound Care*. 1993;2(6):330–336.

Grocott P. The palliative management of fungating malignant wounds. *J Wound Care*. 1995;4(5):240–242.

Mishtriki SK, Jeffery PJ, Law DJW. Wound infection: the surgeon's responsibility. *J Wound Care*. 1992;1(2):32–36.

Müller C, O'Neill A, Mortimer D. Skin problems in palliative care: nursing aspects. In: Doyle D, Hanks G, McDonald N, eds. *Oxford Textbook of Palliative Medicine*. Oxford: Oxford Medical; 1993.

Peplau H. *Interpersonal Relations in Nursing*. New York: GP Putman; 1952.

Roy C, Andrews H. *The Roy Adaptation Model*. 2nd ed. Stamford, CT: Appleton and Lange; 1999.

REFERENCES

1. Coulter A. More active role for patients. *Nursing Standard*. 2000;14(45):5.
2. McQueen A. Nurse-patient relationships and partnerships in hospital care. *J Clin Nurs*. 2000;9(5):723–731.
3. Rodgers SE. The patient facing surgery. In: Alexander MF, Fawcett JN, Runciman PJ, eds. *Nursing Practice*. Edinburgh: Churchill Livingstone; 1999.
4. Smitherman C. *Nursing Actions for Health Promotion*. Philadelphia, PA: FA Davis; 1981.
5. Miller D, Harding K. *Pilonidal Sinus Disease*. World Wide Wounds; 2003. Available at: www.worldwidewounds.com.
6. JU Bascom. Pilonidal sinus. *Curr Pract Surg*. 1994;6:175–180.
7. Senapati A, Cripps NPJ. Pilonidal sinus. In: Johnson CD, Taylor I, eds. *Recent Advances in Surgery 23*. Edinburgh: Churchill Livingstone; 2000.
8. Jones DJ. Pilonidal sinus. *Br Med J*. 1992;305:410–412.
9. Kitchen PRB. Pilonidal sinus: experience with the Karydakis flap. *Br J Surg*. 1996;83:1452–1455.
10. Berry DP. Pilonidal sinus disease. *J Wound Care*. 1992;1(3):29–32.
11. Duxbury MS, Blake SM, Dashfield A, Lambert AW. A randomised trial of knife versus diathermy in pilonidal disease. *Ann R Coll Surg Engl*. 2003;85:405–407

12. Khairi HS, Brown JH. Excision and primary closure of pilonidal sinus. *Ann R Coll Surg Engl*. 1995;77:242–244.
13. Senapati A, Cripps NPJ, Thompson MR. Bascom's operation in the day-surgical management of symptomatic pilonidal sinus. *Br J Surg*. 2000;87:1067–1070.
14. Peterson S, Koch R, Stelzner S. Primary closure techniques in chronic pilonidal sinus. A survey of the results of different surgical approaches. *Dis Colon Rectum*. 2002;45:1458–1467.
15. Cutting KF, White RJ. Criteria for wound infection by indication. In: White RJ, ed. *Trends in Wound Care*. Vol. III. Salisbury: Quay Books; 2004.
16. Thomas J, Paranjothy S. *Royal College of Obstetricians and Gynaecologists Clinical Effectiveness Support Unit. National Sentinel Caesarean Section Audit Report*. London: RCOG Press; 2001.
17. NICE Clinical guidelines 132: cesarean section, 2019. available: https://www.nice.org.uk/guidance/cg132.
18. Orem D. *Nursing – Concepts of Practice*. 5th ed. St Louis, MO: Mosby Yearbook; 1995.
19. Centers for Disease Control and Prevention (CDC). *Wide-ranging online data for epidemiologic research (WONDER)*. Atlanta, GA: CDC, National Center for Health Statistics; 2016. Available at: http://wonder.cdc.gov.
20. Baragwanath P, Shutler S, Harding KG. The management of a patient with a factitious wound. *J Wound Care*. 1994a;3(6):286–287.
21. Purdy, N. (2013). Pastoral Care 11-16: A Critical Introduction, Bloomsbury Publishing.
22. NICE. Clinical. guideline 16: short term physical and psychological management and secondary prevention of self-harm in primary and secondary care; 2004b. Available at: www.nice.org.uk/.
23. Baragwanath P, Gruffudd-Jones A, Young HL, Harding KG. Factitious behaviour in the aetiology of non-healing wounds. In: *Proceedings of the Fourth European Conference on Advances in Wound Management*. London: Macmillan; 1994b.
24. Riehl-Sisca JP. The Riehl interaction model. In: Riehl-Sisca JP, ed. *Conceptual Models for Nursing Practice*. 3rd ed. Norwalk, CT: Appleton and Lange; 1989.

MCQS

1 *Pilonidal sinus wounds are most often seen in young adults. What is the likely causative factor with regard to this age group?*
a. Insufficient hygiene in the wound area
b. Doing too much sport and activities so the tissue is overstretched
c. Unclear, may be related to hormonal changes in the body
d. Infection of fetal tissue

2 *What is the most important aspect of nursing support you can give to a woman after an emergency caesarean?*
a. Organizing help for the baby care
b. Finding a place on the maternity ward for mother and baby
c. Supporting the bonding between mother and child
d. Supporting breastfeeding to help renormalization of the uterus so that the tissue is not overstretched

3 *When considering wound care in young adults in general, which of the following is true?*
   a. They are a generally healthy population with good wound healing potential
   b. Being an active population their special wound care requirements relate to their busy daily routines
   c. Wound healing is prolonged due to a lack of options for immobilizing affected areas
   d. There is no need for wound treatment due to an absence of health issues in this population

Chapter 7

Wound Care in the Middle-Aged Individual

Andrea Pokorná

Highlights

As you read through this chapter concentrate on the following:

- The effect of serious illness and related occurrence of the wound on a previously healthy adult
- The importance of an educative and supportive nursing role
- The use of nurses with special knowledge and skills to complement the care given to patients with wounds
- The importance that underlying disease processes have on wound healing and quality of a patient's life in middle age

Key Issues

This chapter outlines the wound problems encountered by the middle-aged individual. The particular needs of middle-aged patients are described. Attention is paid to the socio-economic situation of patients that affects their treatment, their health literacy and nurses' educative role.

Clinical Case Study

- Aetiology and management of a neuropathic foot ulcer in a man with diabetes mellitus

Nursing Model

- Case study example is viewed through the lens of Peplau's model

Introduction

For many individuals the teenage and adult years are full of activity, parenting and hard work. Middle age can bring financial stability and contentment. There is no sharp physical or psychological demarcation between young and middle adulthood. Developmentalists consider middle adulthood to span the years from 40 to 60 or 65. Cognitive development is at its peak during middle adulthood. The years between 60 to 65 serve as transition years into late adulthood. The period of middle age is usually assumed to begin between the ages of 35 and 45 years and to end at the age of 65 years.[1] When illness happens at this stage of the life cycle, patients can have difficulty accepting it. Malignancy, diabetes mellitus and cardiovascular disease are frequently encountered diseases for this age group.

Diabetic Foot Ulceration

Diabetic foot ulcers are a serious complication of diabetes mellitus. The problem can be compounded by the patient's lifestyle, as in Case Study 7.1.

EPIDEMIOLOGY AND AETIOLOGY

The prevalence of diabetes is on the rise worldwide, especially in developed countries. More than 1 in every 10 adults aged over 18 years is affected.[2] Patients with diabetes are at greater risk of hospitalization compared to the population without diabetes.[3] The incidence of diabetes has more than doubled during the past two decades to a total of 7.2 million hospital discharges, accounting for 43.1 million hospital days among adults in the USA.[2,4] Patients

Case Study 7.1

Diabetic Foot Ulceration

Donald Waites has had insulin-dependent diabetes mellitus for 30 years, having been diagnosed at the age of 25. Following diagnosis of his condition, Donald was very careful in following the advice given and took his insulin according to his blood glucose levels. Patient education was sparse at that time as there were no specialist nurses or clinics, and management was largely controlled by the hospital consultant or GP. As time progressed, like many individuals with diabetes mellitus, Donald began to disregard advice and gave himself extra insulin when going out for a large meal and drinking heavily.

In his 30s and 40s he had many episodes of hypoglycaemia and hyperglycaemia, which on several occasions resulted in admission to hospital. Education regarding diet, weight control and foot care was reinforced on these occasions but by now Donald was becoming resistant to the advice of health professionals, feeling that he had received little support in coping with his condition over the years. These periods of hospitalization resulted in Donald's employment becoming sporadic and he often found himself without work and having to claim unemployment benefit in order to support himself.

Donald, now 55 years old, has been working on a building site as a bricklayer. He is single and has no dependants. Working long hours to claim overtime, he has been continuing to bypass regular meals or insulin. His personal hygiene has also deteriorated and his housing conditions have become squalid.

As far as diabetic management goes, he has not visited his GP for the last 2 years, even though he has been experiencing 'pins and needles' in his arms and hands and a loss of sensation in both feet. This has frightened Donald, as at this time of his life he is fearful of not having employment and being unable to draw a pension.

On return from work yesterday Donald took off his boot and found he had a round ulcer on his right heel. The skin surrounding the wound was red and inflamed and although he could feel nothing, he realized it had been caused by a nail sticking through the heel of his boot. Donald remembered a patient in the bed next to him during his last hospital visit who had had a similar ulcer, and recalled that this man ended up having his leg amputated. Donald went to his doctor the very next morning.

with type 2 diabetes are hospitalized frequently for causes directly related to diabetes complications and stay longer in hospital than those without diabetes.[5] Diabetic foot problems are the cause of more inpatient stays than all other medical problems caused by diabetes.[6] The impact of foot ulceration on an individual's life can be profound, and it is associated with risk of amputation.

As the prevalence of diabetes mellitus and its complications increase rapidly, diabetic foot ulcers (DFUs), which are a major diabetic complication, are expected also to increase. For prevention and effective treatment, it is important to understand the clinical course of DFUs.

Diabetic foot ulceration is the result of a group of syndromes in which neuropathy, ischaemia and infection lead to tissue breakdown; both peripheral neuropathy and peripheral vascular disease can occur simultaneously. It should be highlighted that the depth of the wound and combined infection of DFU, rather than the extent of the wound, are significant prognostic factors of lower extremity amputations (LEAs) in patients with type 2 diabetes.[7]

Neuropathy

Neuropathy is a disease affecting the nerves that causes impairment of sensation, movement and other aspects of health depending upon the nerve affected.[8] Peripheral neuropathy in diabetes is one of the major causes of foot ulcers.[8] Most commonly, peripheral neuropathy affects the lower limbs and can affect sensory, motor or cutaneous nerves. Sensory impairment means that painless neuropathic ulcers can be caused by repeated trauma that the patient is not aware of. For example, this may occur from the pressure and trauma from ill-fitting shoes. Thermal trauma may be caused by the heat of fires or hot-water bottles, which the patient fails to feel. Chemical trauma may result from the diabetic patient applying home remedies, such as over-the-counter treatment for corns, instead of consulting a chiropodist. Patients with neuropathy may cut their toenails too harshly, get sunburnt feet or step on a sharp object without realizing that damage is being done. Neuropathic ulcers are by far the most common cause of diabetic foot ulceration (Fig. 7.1).

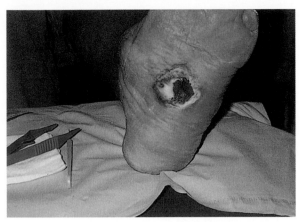

Fig. 7.1 A neuropathic foot ulcer showing Charcot joints of the foot.

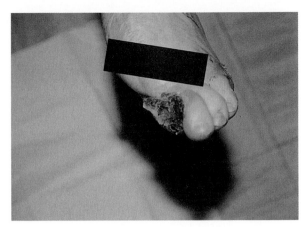

Fig. 7.2 Patient with peripheral vascular disease due to diabetes. The great and first toe have already been amputated due to gangrene.

Peripheral Vascular Disease

Vascular insufficiency affects both large vessels (atherosclerosis) and small vessels (microvascular disease) of the lower limbs in diabetes. Peripheral vascular disease (PVD) is not considered an independent risk factor for DFUs. Rather, it combines with neuropathy and together they are the leading cause of non-traumatic amputations.[9] The distal cells are deprived of the necessary metabolic requirements and the tissues become devitalized. Subsequent injury from ill-fitting footwear can then readily cause ischaemic ulceration of the area (Fig. 7.2).

Thrombosis can also occur, resulting in gangrene of the area supplied by the thrombosed vessel. Thus, gangrene can result from a seemingly minor injury, with very serious consequences. Both life and limb are at risk in this situation. The affected limb, or part of the limb, may require amputation, with infection and septicaemia being potentially lethal.

Identifying the patient at risk of developing foot ulceration is essential if ulceration is to be prevented or damage minimized. The SIGN guidelines in 2010[2] identified risk factors for diabetic patients (Box 7.1).

Many diabetic foot problems can be prevented or the damage minimized through careful monitoring of the patients' feet and effective patient education and self-care promotion. Protective measures are listed in Box 7.2.

ASSESSMENT AND DIAGNOSIS

A full history and examination should be performed relating to the patient's diabetes.[2] If this has already

BOX 7.1 RISK FACTORS FOR DEVELOPING ULCERATION OR GANGRENE

1. Previous ulceration or gangrene
2. Increasing age
3. Peripheral vascular disease
4. Neuropathy
5. Joint deformity
6. Presence of callus
7. Other:
   duration of diabetes
   male sex
   retinopathy
   nephropathy
   visual/mobility problems

From Scottish Intercollegiate Guidelines Network (SIGN). *Management of Diabetes: a National Clinical Guideline*. Edinburgh: Scottish Intercollegiate Guidelines Network; 2010.

been done, accurate documentation should be obtained of the previous history, especially the history of previous DFU or amputation.

Central to the diagnosis is an integrated clinical examination of the foot (Fig. 7.3). All patients with diabetes should be screened to assess their risk of developing a foot ulcer. Patients with active diabetic foot disease should be referred to a multidisciplinary diabetic foot care service. A multidisciplinary foot team should include:

- diabetes nurse specialist
- diabetologist/endocrinologist
- podiatrist
- orthotist

BOX 7.2 MEASURES TO PROTECT THE FEET IN PATIENTS WITH DIABETES MELLITUS[2,8,9,11]

GENERAL MEASURES

- Do not smoke
- Eat a varied and balanced diet to promote good glycaemic control and wound healing
- Exercise; try to keep active. This will help both neuropathy and ischaemia

BASIC FOOT CARE ADVICE

- Try to get shoes that don't pinch anywhere and which allow all toes to move freely. New shoes should never need to be broken in
- Ensure that socks or stockings fit comfortably. Change them daily
- Change footwear as soon as possible if wet
- Avoid walking barefoot; wear slippers and beach shoes to prevent injury
- Bathe feet daily using lukewarm (not hot) water and mild soap
- Pat feet dry gently; pay special attention to the area between the toes

- Apply a moisturizing cream daily (except between the toes) to avoid dryness and keep the skin supple
- Avoid exposing feet to excess heat or cold
- Cut nails to the shape of the end of the toe
- Do not self-treat corns and calluses
- If a minor cut or abrasion does occur, wash thoroughly and cover with a sterile dressing. Seek advice if it has not healed within a few days

SPECIFIC ADVICE FOR PATIENTS WITH NEUROPATHY/ISCHAEMIA

- Inspect feet daily for blisters, corns, calluses, cracks or redness (a mirror can help in seeing the underside of the foot)
- Use of footwear when walking
- Check shoes and socks before putting them on
- Access the foot care service
- Seek advice for treatment of callus from a podiatrist
- Learn the warning signs of infection and other foot problems

From Scottish Intercollegiate Guidelines Network (SIGN). *Management of Diabetes: a National Clinical Guideline*. Edinburgh: Scottish Intercollegiate Guidelines Network; 2010; Shaw JE, Boulton AJM. The pathogenesis of diabetic foot problems: an overview. *Diabetes*. 1997;46(suppl 2):S58–S61; Jeffcoate WJ, Harding KG. Diabetic foot ulcers. *Lancet*. 2003;361(9368):1545–1551; Pendsey SP. Understanding diabetic foot. *Int J Diabetes Dev Ctries*. 2010;30(2):75–79.

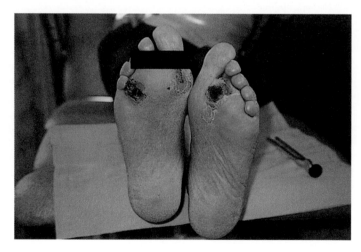

Fig. 7.3 Neuropathic ulcers of both feet. These wounds require debridement of necrotic tissue and callus before wound assessment and care can take place.

- vascular surgeon
- orthopaedic surgeon
- radiologist.

A multidisciplinary foot service should address cardiovascular risk management.[2]

Assessment should aim to:

- ascertain the type, onset and duration of diabetes
- identify current or developing complications of diabetes (especially occurrence of hypo- or hyperglycaemia)
- diagnose the exact nature and aetiology of the ulcer (differentiate the type of ulcer)
- prescribe the correct medical or surgical treatment

- identify suitable dressing and foot care that will enhance healing.

Important points to be recorded are summarized in Table 7.1,[2-4,10] while Table 7.2[11] lists the clinical features that differentiate neuropathic and ischemic ulceration. The classic diabetic trophic ulcer must be also distinguished from various other problems that tend to occur in persons with diabetes, such as diabetic dermopathy, bullosis diabeticorum, eruptive xanthoma, necrobiosis lipoidica and granuloma annulare. The leg pain of peripheral arterial disease must be distinguished from other causes of leg pain, such as arthritis, muscle pain, radicular pain, spinal cord compression, thrombophlebitis, anaemia and myxoedema.

Specific Examinations (see also Chapter 9)

For Ischaemia

Palpation of pedal pulses is not a reliable indicator for the assessment of ischaemia and should not be used. To confirm the presence of pulses and to quantify the vascular supply a Doppler ultrasonographic assessment should be done. Instructions of how to do a Doppler ultrasonographic assessment as well as how to measure the ankle–brachial pressure index (ABPI) or ankle–brachial index (ABI) and a table with the interpretation of the results are outlined in Chapter 9.

Be aware: Patients with diabetes mellitus may give falsely high (i.e., normal) readings owing to calcification of the arteries so they should always be viewed with caution and in conjunction with a full medical history. In specialist units, other more in-depth vascular assessments may be carried out, such as transcutaneous oxygen tension (TcPO$_2$) with abnormal value less than 40 mmHg and plethysmography or absolute toe systolic pressure (abnormal value less than 45 mmHg).

For Neuropathy

The vibration threshold can be measured using a biothesiometer; vibrations can be transmitted through the patient's foot to indicate the extent of sensory loss. Simpler measurements using a 128-Hz tuning fork or a 10-g Semmes-Weinstein monofilament can be performed by any practitioner. If these are not available,

TABLE 7.1 Important Facts to be Ascertained in Patients with Diabetic Ulceration

Record	Rationale
Date of birth	Age is a risk factor for PVD
Sex	PVD and amputations are more common in men
Type of diabetes and treatment	Methods of achieving good control. May change treatment if control poor
Duration of diabetes	Prevalence of neuropathy and ischaemia increase with diabetes duration
History of ischaemic heart disease, myocardial infarctions, cerebrovascular accident, angina	Indication of arteriosclerosis and ischaemia
Smoking, hyperlipidaemia, obesity	Risk factor for PVD in diabetic patients
Compliance	Key factor in aetiology of ulcer and aftercare management
History of intermittent claudication	Indicative of ischaemia
Rest pain	
Previous arterial surgery	

PVD, Peripheral vascular disease.
From Scottish Intercollegiate Guidelines Network (SIGN). *Management of Diabetes: a National Clinical Guideline.* Edinburgh: Scottish Intercollegiate Guidelines Network; 2010; Donnan P, Leese G, Morris A, Diabetes Audit and Research in Tayside, Scotland/Medicine Monitoring Unit Collaboration. Hospitalizations for people with type 1 and type 2 diabetes compared with the nondiabetic population of Tayside, Scotland: A retrospective cohort study of resource use. *Diabetes Care,* 2000;23(12):1774–1779, National Diabetes Statistics Report. Atlanta: Centers for Disease Control and Prevention; 2017; Rasmussen A, Almdal T, Anker et al. Decreasing incidence of foot ulcer among patients with type 1 and type 2 diabetes in the period 2001–2014. *Diabetes Res Clin Pract.* 2017;130:221–228.

TABLE 7.2   Differential Diagnosis of Neuropathic and Ischaemic Ulceration

Clinical Feature	Neuropathic Foot	Ischaemic Foot
Colour	Normal or red appearance indicating cellulitis or early Charcot foot	Pale/cyanotic Rubor on dependency; blanches on elevation (Buerger's test)
Deformity	Claw toe Hammer toe Charcot deformity	Nil Absent toes from previous surgery
Callus tissue	Found on plantar surface of metatarsal head/apices or toes	Nil – thin skin
Tissue breakdown	Ulcers commonly found on plantar surface	Ulcers commonly found on the margins Visible signs of digital gangrene
Peripheral pulses	Present (may be difficult to palpate if swollen or deformed foot)	Dorsalis pedis and/or posterior tibial absent May not be absent if small vessel disease
Temperature	Feels normal or warm	Feels cold
Skin moisture	Dry foot Decrease in perspiration	Normal
Sensation	Impaired sensation to pinprick/light touch, position and vibration	Normal
Tendon reflex	Impaired	Normal

From Pendsey SP. Understanding diabetic foot. *Int J Diabetes Dev Ctries*. 2010;30(2):75–79.

the detection of light touch by cotton wool, pinprick and vibration sense using a 128-Hz tuning fork is sufficient. The goal is to detect whether the patient has loss of protective sensations (LOPS), rendering him/her susceptible to foot ulceration.[11] Magnetic resonance imaging (MRI) can be used to detect early changes of Charcot neuroarthropathy, which cannot be identified by X-ray.

Other Examinations

Retinal examination indicates the absence or degree of retinopathy. Other investigations are listed in Table 7.3.

SCREENING

During annual foot screening, patients should receive verbal and written advice on the following:
- how diabetes affects their feet
- why it is important to have foot screening and risk assessment

TABLE 7.3   Other Investigations in Diabetic Foot Ulceration

Record	Rationale
Haemoglobin (HbA1c)	Good measure of long-term control
Urea and creatinine	Measurement of renal function indicative of nephropathy
Proteinuria	Indicative of nephropathy
Wound swab	Confirms clinical signs of infection

- how to care for their feet and when to seek help
- how to contact podiatry services within working hours
- what to do in an emergency out of hours
- patients could be offered NHS Scotland leaflets on low, moderate or high risk of non-healing

TABLE 7.4 Assessment of Donald's Problems (Case Study 7.1)	
Subjective Experience of Patient	**Objective Observation by Nurse**
Little faith in health professionals Not wanting to be labelled as ill	Patient non-compliant with treatment Patient unaware of health status
Feels he can control illness by altering insulin according to social needs	Little understanding of the pathology of the disease process
Frightened of the consequences of his complaint	Has not reported signs of neuropathy until ulcer developed Displaying signs of advanced disease process
Frightened that ulceration could lead to amputation	Localized infection in and around ulcer, possibility of invasive infection
Does not understand why he did not feel nail in shoe rubbing	Not aware of signs of diabetic neuropathy Does not inspect feet daily
Finds it increasingly difficult to keep up with personal hygiene and domestic chores	Looks unkempt; nobody at home to provide support
Worried that period of sickness will result in unemployment	Financial difficulties due to sporadic employment

wounds and amputation (all available from http://www.diabetesinscotland.org.uk). These leaflets should only be provided after screening and should be part of their management plan

- other NHS Scotland foot advice leaflets as appropriate, e.g., *Footwear advice to reduce the risk of amputation; Advice to help you care for your feet on holiday* (also from http://www.diabetesinscotland.org.uk).

MANAGEMENT

The diabetic foot should be managed using a multi-disciplinary team approach as mentioned earlier. Foot care education is recommended as part of a multidisciplinary approach in all patients with diabetes.

Healing is likely to be impaired in the patient with diabetes mellitus as there is a reduction in the inflammatory response and granulation tissue formation. Neuropathic ulcers usually take weeks or months to heal, even with the appropriate resources. Some patients require complete bed rest combined with removal of weight bearing and friction. For patients with ischaemic ulcers, reconstructive arterial surgery should always be considered, although the optimum time for this to happen is difficult to determine.[2]

Feet and Charcot Foot - Treatment and Management

Patients at high risk of ulceration or amputation, or who have previously had ulceration or amputation should be provided with a management plan prepared with their input. Those who present with no risk factors should be given advice regarding self-care and self-management.

Active Foot Disease

Patients with active foot ulceration should be referred to a multidisciplinary foot care service for the following advice and information:

- multidisciplinary foot care service emergency contact details
- emergency out of hours contact details
- risk factor modification, e.g. smoking cessation and good glycaemic control
- wound care and antibiotics, when required
- appropriate off-loading
- complications as a result of therapy
- relevant patient support leaflets, e.g., *Looking after your foot ulcer; Advice for looking after your Charcot foot* (available from http://www.diabetesinscotland.org.uk).

General issues related to the disease process of diabetes mellitus should be considered, i.e., control of the disease and referral to the appropriate specialist for reconstructive surgery or medical treatment of complications. Continuing care and maintenance of the foot can be given, ideally at a multidisciplinary foot clinic or by a chiropodist/podiatrist. Nail and foot care can be provided and problems detected at an early stage.

Ideally all weight should be relieved from the ulcerated area and redistributed. This can be achieved by an orthotist designing and making footwear for the patient. There is limited evidence that padded hosiery can reduce peak plantar pressures. In contrast, patients who routinely wear their prescription shoes and orthoses are less likely to have ulcer relapse.[12]

Daily inspection of the feet by the patient should be undertaken, regardless of whether the foot is ulcerated or not. Any signs of redness, heat, blistering or bleeding should be looked for and immediate treatment sought. If ignored, the foot could rapidly deteriorate and lead to invasive infection of the limb.

Dressings useful for the treatment of foot ulceration include absorbent foams, which act as padding and protection for the injured area. For moderate or heavily exuding ulcers, alginate dressings can provide absorbency without too much bulk. Semi-occlusive dressings such as hydrocolloids or adhesive dressings that are not changed daily – and so prevent daily foot inspection – are best avoided.

Regular debridement of callus build-up around the ulcer bed is advised. All callus, or as much as possible, should be removed to prevent further trauma to the area.

Patient education is of paramount importance in the prevention and/or deterioration of foot ulcers. Education will help to empower the patient to take control of their condition and minimize complications.

Negative-pressure wound therapy should be considered in patients with active diabetic foot ulcers or postoperative wounds. All patients with critical limb ischaemia, including rest pain, ulceration and tissue loss, should be considered for arterial reconstruction.

Opiate analgesia in combination with gabapentin should be considered for the treatment of patients with diabetic painful neuropathy that cannot be controlled with monotherapy.[2]

The following aspects of management are key for the treatment and prevention of DFUs and their complications:

Patient Education

Education on foot care, as well as on the control of blood sugar levels, should be undertaken at an early stage. This can also be done with the aid of diabetic educators, district nurses and social workers.

Blood Sugar Control

This is managed using a team approach of GP, diabetologist/diabetes nurse and vascular specialist, and is based on the severity of the disease (according to an appropriate assessment tool) and the patient's attitude towards medication, especially insulin.

Decreasing Pressure

Preventing further or new trauma by off-loading pressure to the area can be done with crutches, wheelchairs or casting. Ulcer healing is improved with total contact casting or irremovable cast walkers (in contrast to removable cast walkers).

Improving Peripheral Vascular Circulation

Antiplatelet agents are the initial drug therapy; however, insufficiency requires surgical bypass.

Prevention or Control of Infection

Systemic and source control is achieved using antibiotics and surgical debridement.

Topical Ulcer Care

Principles of wound care include the use of topical agents with dressing and debridement.

Nursing Model for Donald

Having visited his GP, who performed a full assessment (Table 7.4), Donald was diagnosed as having a neuropathic foot ulcer. The GP transferred wound care to the district nurse. If the district nurse uses Peplau's model, consider what particular aspects of the model are pertinent to assessing and planning Donald's care? Note that Table 7.4 addresses the 'S' (subjective experience of the patient) and 'O' (objective observation made by nurse) of the SOAP acronym. Table 7.5 then addresses 'A' (assessment and identification of problems) and 'P' (plan of action).

Development models often focus on the educative-counselling role the nurse plays. This is of paramount importance, as often the care a patient needs may be different from what they want. Do you think that Donald wants the care and advice

TABLE 7.5 Identification of Problems in Table 7.4 and Plan of Action

Identification of Problem	Plan of Action
Infected neuropathic ulcer	Debridement of ulcer by doctor, nurse specialist or chiropodist Dressing with absorbent dressing (foam or alginate), wound cleansing with saline to remove dressing material – dressing changes according the amount of exudate Swab to identify infecting organism; initially treat with broad-spectrum antibiotic orally One-week period of non-weight bearing
Poor understanding of diet and diabetic control	Diabetic specialist nurse and community dietician to visit patient at home District nurse to reinforce information with patient education programme
Long-term history of unstable diabetes	Assessment of HbA1c blood test Renal function, eye retinopathy, extent of neuropathy Referral to special centre with multidisciplinary team
Lack of knowledge concerning care of feet	District nurse to explain importance of inspection of feet daily, hygiene and clean footwear Refer to orthotist for removal of friction Refer to chiropodist
Reluctant to seek support of health professionals	District nurse to promote a trusting relationship with patient by listening to his point of view Planning care together with realistic goals – finding a common solution Introducing other specialists to patients at separate intervals Collecting and evaluating all the information to inform patient
Lives alone, no social support	Encourage patient to join local diabetic association; find out details of local group
Fear of loss of employment and lack of secure income	Arrange visit of social worker to reassess benefit entitlement Consider change of employment to less manual work

HbA1c, haemoglobin A1c.

the district nurse is going to give? (Probably he does not.)

Peplau's philosophy of nursing stresses the importance of the formation of the relationship between nurse and patient. The first purpose of the nurse is to minimize or remove the risks to the patient's health but the second is to help the individual to understand and come to terms with their health problem. In Donald's case this will require a great deal of input. However, this is at the core of person-centred care for all patients, including those with diabetes.

Practice Point

Donald Waites' case stresses the importance of the nurse's role in helping patients to understand and come to terms with their condition.

Summary

Two essential aspects for the provision of high-level wound care for middle-aged patients are highlighted in this chapter.

- The transition from health to serious illness in an adult requires the nurse to function in an educative role with respect to a patient's socio-cultural background.
- There is a key role for nurses with special knowledge and skills who give a high level of professional care to their patients.

If you work with any specialist practitioners, observe the skills they use to enhance patient care. Be aware of the need for multidisciplinary and team working and comprehensive person-centred care.

FURTHER READING

Bryant RA, Nix DP. *Acute and Chronic Wounds: Current Management Concepts.* 5th ed. St. Louis, MO: Elsevier; 2016.

Nather A. *Diabetic Foot Problems.* Singapore: World Scientific Publishing Co.; 2008.

Piaggesi A, Apelqvist J, eds. *The Diabetic Foot Syndrome.* Basel: S. Karger; 2017.

Stryja J, Sandy-Hodgetts K, Collier M, Moser K, Ousey K, Probst S, Wilson J, Xuereb D. Surgical site infection: preventing and managing surgical site infection across health care sectors. *J Wound Care.* 2020;29:2, (Suppl. 2):S1–S69

REFERENCES

1. Barclay SR, Stoltz KB, Chung YB. Voluntary midlife career change: integrating the transtheoretical model and the life-span, life-space approach. *Career Dev Q.* 2011;59(5):386–399.
2. Scottish Intercollegiate Guidelines Network (SIGN). *Management of Diabetes: a National Clinical Guideline.* Edinburgh: Scottish Intercollegiate Guidelines Network; 2010.
3. Donnan P, Leese G, Morris A. Diabetes Audit and Research in Tayside, Scotland/Medicine Monitoring Unit Collaboration. Hospitalizations for people with type 1 and type 2 diabetes compared with the nondiabetic population of Tayside, Scotland: a retrospective cohort study of resource use. *Diabetes Care.* 2000;23(12):1774–1779.
4. *National Diabetes Statistics Report.* Atlanta: Centers for Disease Control and Prevention; 2017.
5. Khalid JM, Raluy-Callado M, Curtis BH, Boye KS, Maguire A, Reaney M. Rates and risk of hospitalisation among patients with type 2 diabetes: retrospective cohort study using the UK General Practice Research Database linked to English Hospital Episode Statistics. *Int J Clin Pract.* 2014;68(1):40–48.
6. Comino EJ, Harris MF, Islam MDF, et al. Impact of diabetes on hospital admission and length of stay among a general population aged 45 year or more: a record linkage study. *BMC Health Services Res.* 2015;15:12.
7. Jeong EG, Cho SS, Lee SH, et al. Depth and combined infection is important predictor of lower extremity amputations in hospitalized diabetic foot ulcer patients. *Korean J Intern Med.* 2018;33(5):952–960.
8. Shaw JE, Boulton AJM. The pathogenesis of diabetic foot problems: an overview. *Diabetes.* 1997;46(suppl 2):S58–S61.
9. Jeffcoate WJ, Harding KG. Diabetic foot ulcers. *Lancet.* 2003;361(9368):1545–1551.
10. Rasmussen A, Almdal T, Anker Nielsen A, et al. Decreasing incidence of foot ulcer among patients with type 1 and type 2 diabetes in the period 2001–2014. *Diabetes Res Clin Pract.* 2017;130:221–228.
11. Pendsey SP. Understanding diabetic foot. *Int J Diabetes Dev Ctries.* 2010;30(2):75–79.
12. Richardson CR, Mehari KS, McIntyre LG, et al. A randomized trial comparing structured and lifestyle goals in an internet-mediated walking program for people with type 2 diabetes. *Int J Behav Nutrition Phy Act.* 2007;4:59.

MCQS

1 *A structured screening programme in patients with diabetes should result in:*
  a. Prevention and early detection of ulceration
  b. An increase in the incidence of major amputation
  c. An increase in the hospitalization rates
  d. A decreased incidence of major amputation

2 *In diabetic patients with active foot ulceration, do vacuum-assisted wound closure devices/negative-pressure wound therapy (NPWT) devices improve healing outcomes?*
  a. Yes, NPWT should be considered in all patients with active DFU or postoperative wounds
  b. Yes, NPWT should be considered in patients with active DFU or postoperative wounds as an adjunct to standard wound care on an individual level
  c. No, NPWT is not suggested for patients with DFU
  d. There is not enough evidence to support NPWT in patients with DFU and its effect is not clear

3 *Which of the following debridement techniques should be used as a first step to improve healing outcomes in diabetic patients with active foot ulceration?*
  a. Surgical debridement
  b. Biosurgical (larval) debridement
  c. Local sharp debridement
  d. Hydrojet therapy – 'versajet'

4 *Which of the following is an* **extrinsic** *risk factor for the development of surgical site infections in patients with active DFU?*
  a. Emergency nature of surgery
  b. Diabetes
  c. Tobacco use
  d. Malnutrition

Chapter 8

Pressure Ulcers and Incontinence-Associated Dermatitis in Older Individuals

Dimitri Beeckman and Brecht Serraes

Highlights

As you read through this chapter concentrate on the following:

- Recognition of the predisposing factors that contribute to pressure ulcer (PU) development and incontinence-associated dermatitis (IAD)
- Use of the appropriate risk assessment methods to assess patients
- Selection of materials, products and procedures to adequately prevent PUs and IAD
- Involvement of the multidisciplinary team in the delivery of care
- Differentiation of PU from IAD using PuClas guidelines
- Classification of PU and IAD using an appropriate classification system

Key Issues

This chapter deals with skin and tissue integrity issues, pressure ulcers (PUs) and incontinence-associated dermatitis (IAD), in older individuals, which are associated with immobility and incontinence issues.

Clinical Case Study

Prevention of PUs and IAD in an older individual in a nursing home setting

Introduction

The world's population is ageing; virtually every country in the world is experiencing growth in the number and proportion of older persons in their population. According to data from the 2017 Revision of the World Population Prospects, the number of older persons – those aged 60 years or more – is expected to more than double by 2050 and to more than triple by 2100. This means that numbers will be rising from 962 million globally in 2017 to 2.1 billion in 2050 and 3.1 billion in 2100. Globally, the population aged 60 or over is growing faster than all younger age groups.[1]

The key characteristics in ageing are increased risk of multimorbidity, a decrease in physical performance, and care dependency. In addition, advanced age, chronic and acute diseases and treatments (e.g. polypharmacy) lead, either directly or indirectly, to a wide range of skin and tissue problems. Pressure ulcers (PUs) and incontinence-associated dermatitis (IAD) are some of the most prevalent skin and tissue problems in geriatric settings.

Examples of problems associated with increasing age include:

- multimorbidity
- decrease of physical performance
- changes in metabolic processes
- continence issues, increased risk of falling, cognitive disorders (such as dementia and Alzheimer's disease)
- lack of medical resources due to financial constraints
- loneliness and social isolation.

BOX 8.1 GLOSSARY

Bulla:
A circumscribed lesion >1 cm in diameter that contains clear, serous or haemorrhagic liquid; a large blister.

Erosion:
Loss of either a portion of or the entire epidermis.

Excoriation:
A loss of the epidermis and a portion of the dermis due to scratching or an exogenous injury.

Maceration:
An appearance or surface softening due to constant wetting – frequently white.

Papule:
An elevated, solid, palpable lesion that is ≤1 cm in diameter.

Pustule:
A circumscribed lesion that contains pus.

Scale:
A visible accumulation of keratin, forming a flat plate or flake.

Swelling:
Enlargement due to accumulation of oedema or fluid, including blood.

Vesicle:
A circumscribed lesion ≤1 cm in diameter that contains clear, serous or haemorrhagic liquid; a small blister.

Common and usually interrelated conditions such as impaired mobility, delirium, frailty, malnutrition, incontinence or falls are often summarized as 'geriatric syndrome'. This is a unique feature in this aged vulnerable population. A glossary of dermatology terms that are used to describe and classify PUs and IAD are given in Box 8.1.

Pressure Ulcers

PUs and IAD are a growing problem in the ageing population and can easily arise in the situation described in Case Study 8.1.

EPIDEMIOLOGY

A systematic review by Hahnel et al. reported the incidence and prevalence rates of skin conditions in the aged population worldwide. A PU prevalence ranging from 0.3% to 46% and a PU incidence from 0.8% to 34% were identified.[2] The majority of these epidemiological data were reported for hospitals (38.7%) and institutional long-term care settings (29.7%), limiting our knowledge about the occurrence of PUs in populations living in the community.[2] According to the clinical practice guideline for PU prevention and treatment published in 2014 and summarizing prevalence and incidence rates reported in the literature between January 2000 to December 2012, prevalence rates in the aged care setting range from 4.1% to 32.2% versus incidence rates ranging from 1.9% to 59%. Prevalence rates in the acute setting (0% to 46%) and critical care setting (13.1% to 45.5%) even seem to be higher compared to that in aged care. Incidence rates in the acute setting range from 0% to 12% and in critical care from 3.3% to 53.4%.[3] In 2008, Vanderwee et al. conducted a PU point prevalence study in 48 Belgian hospitals (n = 19,968 patients), revealing an overall prevalence of category I–IV PUs of 12.1%.[4] The prevalence of category II, III and IV PUs was 3.6%, 2.5% and 1.6%, respectively.[5] In 2012, a PU point prevalence study was conducted in 84 Flemish nursing homes (n = 8008 residents). Comparable prevalence rates were obtained for category II, III and IV PUs (2.9%, 1.9% and 1.1%, respectively).[5]

The wide variations in prevalence and incidence rates are caused by differences in methodological design and rigor of epidemiological studies. It is therefore recommended to describe, among other things, PU rates within various PU risk levels and common anatomical locations of PU and to differentiate PUs by category, clearly indicating whether category I PUs were included or excluded in the final calculations.[3]

The costs associated with PUs are considerable. According to the Agency for Healthcare Research & Quality (AHRQ), PUs cost the US healthcare system between $9.1 billion and $11.6 billion annually. In addition to direct treatment-related costs, PUs also result in litigation and government penalties, and impact hospital performance metrics. Demarré et al. systematically reviewed the evidence of the cost of preventing and treating PUs across all settings. Not surprisingly, the cost of PU treatment was found to be greater than the cost of prevention. The cost per patient per day ranged between €1.71 and €470.49 for treatment and between €2.65 and €87.57 for prevention, across all settings. The cost of prevention in long-term care settings (e.g., nursing homes) per patient per day ranged between €2.65 and €19.69.[6] On top of the financial implications, PUs also have a significant impact on patient morbidity, mortality and

Case Study 8.1

Pressure Ulcers and Incontinence-Associated Dermatitis

Elsie Mason is an 83-year-old woman who, for the past 6 years, has been in residential care in a nursing home as her husband found it increasingly difficult to cope. Initially admitted for bouts of forgetfulness and inability to care for herself, her psychological condition has deteriorated dramatically over the last 2 years and she has recently been diagnosed as having Alzheimer's disease. Whereas previously Elsie had been fairly mobile, she has recently been difficult to mobilize and spends long periods in bed, often missing meals. She has also become incontinent of urine and faeces, failing to indicate to the staff when she wants to go to the toilet. She is often found wandering around at night and is becoming increasingly difficult to communicate with. Her husband is most distressed with her deterioration, especially as she often does not recognize him and tells people he is dead. Three weeks ago, while Elsie was being bathed, a small red area was noticed on her left hip. Although this was thought insignificant at the time, within 4 days the whole of the hip had become blackened and lost the outer skin covering. Two weeks later a larger cavity 12 cm × 10.2 cm and 2 cm in depth appeared. Additionally, she developed a large area of inflammation in the perigenital area associated with skin loss (denudation) and clinical signs of a secondary fungal infection.

quality of life.[7–9] To further exacerbate the problem, as the population ages, the percentage of patients at risk for developing PUs is growing, thus increasing the demand for early-stage prevention.

AETIOLOGY

A PU is defined as 'a localized injury to the skin and/or underlying tissue, usually over a bony prominence, resulting from sustained pressure (including pressure associated with shear)'.[3] PUs are caused by a sustained mechanical load in the form of pressure or pressure and shear, causing deformation of skin and subdermal tissues (fat tissue, connective tissue and muscles). Consequently, strain (i.e., a measure of relative deformation) and stress (i.e., force transferred per unit area) within the tissues occur, which can hinder transport processes within the tissues.[3]

It is recognized that both the magnitude and the time duration are important in the development of PUs.[10] As a result, both a high load applied for a short period and a low load applied for a prolonged period can lead to tissue damage.[11–17] The nature of the mechanical load (i.e., pressure, shear and friction) is of importance when analyzing the mechanical boundary conditions as it also has an impact on the internal strains and stresses (Fig. 8.1).[10] *Pressure* can be defined as a force perpendicular to the skin surface, in contrast to *shear*, where forces are moving parallel and in opposite directions to the skin surface.[3] Shear is a result of a combination of friction and gravity. *Friction* is the force of two surfaces rubbing against one another (e.g., the feet of a restless patient rubbing across the bed sheets).[18]

Additionally, the mechanical properties of the tissue, the geometry of the tissue and the underlying bones, the individual transport (perfusion and lymphatic drainage) and thermal properties, and the individual physiology and repair capacity have an impact on the susceptibility and tolerance of the individual for PU development.[10] Ischaemia and deformation are

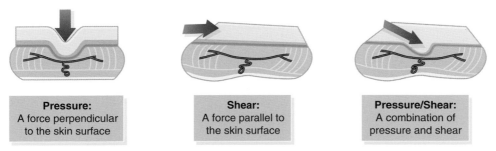

| Pressure: A force perpendicular to the skin surface | Shear: A force parallel to the skin surface | Pressure/Shear: A combination of pressure and shear |

Fig. 8.1 The forces of pressure and shear on the skin and underlying tissues.

well-studied mechanisms leading to the development of tissue damage.[3] Ischaemia is caused by obstruction or occlusion of the blood vessels in soft tissues due to sustained external loading[13,14,19–21] and results in hypoxia, reduced supply of nutrients to cells, reduced elimination of metabolites and a change in pH. The maximum period that ischaemia can be tolerated without damage depends on the mechanical properties of the tissue. Because muscle tissue and fat tissue are less stiff than skin tissue, these are more susceptible to damage.[16,22–26] Based on animal studies, the first signs of ischaemic damage in muscle tissues can be found after 2 hours of sustained pressure.[13,19–21,24,27,28] After off-loading, the degree of tissue damage may be aggravated by reperfusion, because this involves the release of harmful oxygen free radicals.[29–34]

Furthermore, when strains exceeding a critical threshold are applied to the tissue, the resulting deformation can lead to immediate tissue damage, possibly through a direct rupture of the cytoskeleton, stretching of the plasma membrane or internal pathways causing cell death.[11,12,17,35–37] In this case, the extent of tissue damage is determined by the duration of the exposure.[38]

CLASSIFICATION

PUs can start superficially or deep within the tissues, depending on the nature of the surface loading and the tissue integrity. Superficial ulcers form within the skin and may progress downward, whereas deep ulcers arise in muscle layers covering bony prominences and are mainly caused by sustained compression of these tissues.[37–39] The severity of PUs vary from non-blanchable erythema of intact skin to tissue destruction involving skin, subcutaneous fat, muscle and bone. In 1989 the US National Pressure Ulcer Advisory Panel (NPUAP) developed a classification using four stages. This classification system was adopted in Europe in 1999 by the European Pressure Ulcer Advisory Panel (EPUAP) with some minor textual changes.[40] From 2009 onwards, NPUAP and EPUAP developed a common international classification system for PUs. The purpose of the classification system is to standardize record keeping and provide a common description of ulcer severity for the purposes of clinical practice, audit and research.[41] Box 8.2 presents the 2014 NPUAP/EPUAP International Pressure Ulcer Classification system.[3]

RISK ASSESSMENT

The first step in PU prevention is identifying patients at risk. During the last decades, more than 100 factors increasing the probability of PU development have been described and extensively reviewed. However, a (statistical) association between a patient characteristic and PU development does not necessarily indicate a causal relationship. Based on our current understanding, immobility, skin and tissue alterations, and poor perfusion directly cause PUs. Many other variables increase the susceptibility to pressure ulceration, but only if the direct causal factors are present. Among others, these are diabetes mellitus, cachexia, acute illness, frailty and increased skin surface moisture.

Advanced chronological age can also be considered to be an indirect PU risk factor; that is, nobody gets a pressure ulcer because he/she is old, but rather old age is associated with various changes making the individual more susceptible. For instance, there is an age-associated increase in skin and tissue stiffening and a slower recovery after deformation. The stiffer a soft tissue, the higher the shear loads, and the larger is the susceptibility to deformation injury. At sun-protected areas, skin ageing is associated with an increase in skin roughness. Increased skin surface roughness may lead to an increased coefficient of friction leading to higher shear loads in the skin. Diminished perfusion and innate immune response and a flattening of the dermo–epidermal junction further contribute to higher PU risk in aged patients. Advanced age and the presence of frailty are always strongly associated with poor health and limited mobility, which in turn is the strongest predictor for PU development. This is the reason for the many well-known associations between geriatric assessment measures and PUs – these include handgrip strength and PUs, malnutrition and PUs, and between PU risk measures and care dependency or mortality in geriatric populations.

During risk assessment, the above-mentioned risk factors must be considered and a comprehensive head-to-toe skin assessment must be conducted focusing on PU predilection areas. Special emphasis should be put on the assessment of activity, mobility, existing PUs or other skin alterations such as the presence of IAD. During the last decades, numerous standardized PU risk assessment scales have been introduced and are used worldwide. The consensus is that while such scales

BOX 8.2 NPUAP/EPUAP INTERNATIONAL PRESSURE ULCER CLASSIFICATION SYSTEM

Category/Stage I: Non-blanchable Erythema

Intact skin with non-blanchable redness of a localized area usually over a bony prominence. Darkly pigmented skin may not have visible blanching; its colour may differ from the surrounding area. The area may be painful, firm, soft, warmer or cooler as compared to adjacent tissue. Category/Stage I may be difficult to detect in individuals with dark skin tones. May indicate 'at risk' individuals (a heralding sign of risk).

Category/Stage II: Partial-Thickness Skin Loss

Partial-thickness loss of dermis presenting as a shallow, open ulcer with a red-pink wound bed, without slough. May also present as an intact or open/ruptured serum-filled blister. Presents as a shiny or dry shallow ulcer without slough or bruising.* This category/stage should not be used to describe skin tears, tape burns, perineal dermatitis, maceration or excoriation.

Category/Stage III: Full-Thickness Skin Loss

Full-thickness tissue loss. Subcutaneous fat may be visible but bone, tendon or muscle are not exposed. Slough may be present but does not obscure the depth of tissue loss. May include undermining and tunnelling. The depth of a category/stage III pressure ulcer varies by anatomical location. The bridge of the nose, ear, occiput and malleolus do not have subcutaneous tissue and category/stage III ulcers can be shallow. In contrast, areas of significant adiposity can develop extremely deep category/stage III PUs. Bone/tendon is not visible or directly palpable.

Category/Stage IV: Full-Thickness Tissue Loss

Full-thickness tissue loss with exposed bone, tendon or muscle. Slough or eschar may be present on some parts of the wound bed. Often include undermining and tunnelling. The depth of a category/stage IV pressure ulcer varies by anatomical location. The bridge of the nose, ear, occiput and malleolus do not have subcutaneous tissue and these ulcers can be shallow. Category/stage IV ulcers can extend into muscle and/or supporting structures (e.g., fascia, tendon or joint capsule) making osteomyelitis possible. Exposed bone/tendon is visible or directly palpable.

Unstageable: Depth Unknown

Full-thickness tissue loss in which the base of the ulcer is covered by slough (yellow, tan, grey, green or brown) and/or eschar (tan, brown or black) in the wound bed. Until enough slough and/or eschar is removed to expose the base of the wound, the true depth, and therefore category/stage, cannot be determined. Stable (dry, adherent, intact without erythema or fluctuance) eschar on the heels serves as 'the body's natural (biological) cover' and should not be removed.

Suspected Deep-Tissue Injury: Depth Unknown

Purple or maroon localized area of discoloured intact skin or blood-filled blister due to damage of underlying soft tissue from pressure and/or shear. The area may be preceded by tissue that is painful, firm, mushy, boggy, warmer or cooler as compared to adjacent tissue. Deep tissue injury may be difficult to detect in individuals with dark skin tones. Evolution may include a thin blister over a dark wound bed. The wound may further evolve and become covered by thin eschar. Evolution may be rapid, exposing additional layers of tissue even with optimal treatment.

*Bruising indicates suspected deep tissue injury.

Reproduced with permission from NPUAP/EPUAP/PPPIA. Prevention and Treatment of Pressure Ulcers: Clinical Practice Guideline. Osborne Park, Australia: Cambridge Media; 2014.

may be used, obtained scores alone are insufficient for clinical decision making. If risk assessment tools are selected as a structured approach for risk assessment, additional factors (e.g., perfusion, skin status and other relevant risks) should be considered as part of a comprehensive risk assessment. Regardless of how the risk assessment is structured, clinical judgment is essential. Based on international guidelines, the following procedure is recommended:[3]

- Use a structured approach to risk assessment that includes assessment of activity/mobility and skin status.
  - Consider bedfast and/or chairfast individuals to be at risk of PU development.
  - Consider the impact of mobility limitations on PU risk.
- Complete a comprehensive risk assessment for bedfast and/or chairfast individuals to guide preventive interventions.
- Consider individuals with a category/stage I PU to be at risk of progression or new category/stage II and greater PUs.
- Consider individuals with an existing PU (any category/stage) to be at risk of additional PUs.
- Consider the general status of skin on PU risk.
- Consider the impact of the following factors on an individual's risk of PU development:
  - perfusion and oxygenation
  - poor nutritional status
  - increased skin moisture.
- Consider the potential impact of the following factors on an individual's risk of PU development:

- increased body temperature
- advanced age
- sensory perception
- haematological measurements
- general health status.

PREVENTION

The aim of PU prevention is to reduce the duration and/or the amount of pressure and shear. Since preventive measures are expensive and labour intensive,[42] patients with a clear risk of developing PUs should be identified through a structured risk assessment. The prevention of PUs comprises: (1) the use of adequate support surfaces (bed and chair) to redistribute pressure/shear and to manage tissue load and microclimate,[3,43] (2) preventive skin care including cleansing the skin and protecting it from exposure to moisture and (3) systematic repositioning of the patient with consideration of the individual's situation.[43,44]

A support surface is a specialized device for pressure redistribution that is designed for the management of tissue loads, microclimate and/or other therapeutic functions.[45] There is a wide variety of specialized devices available with different product characteristics, e.g., mattresses, integrated bed systems, mattress overlays, seat cushions and seat cushion overlays. These have a range of pressure-redistribution mechanisms for the prevention and treatment of PUs, including: (1) redistributing the weight over the maximum body surface area based on the principles of immersion and envelopment; (2) mechanically alternating the pressure beneath the body to reduce the duration of the applied pressure to each area; (3) a combination of (1) and (2), allowing healthcare professionals to change the mode according to individual needs of the person (Table 8.1).[18,45–49] Considering most PUs could be prevented, there are still not enough resources allocated to provide the necessary emphasis towards prevention.

Patient repositioning must take into account the condition of the patient and the support surface in use.[3,43,44] Specific devices should be placed to elevate (off-load) the heel so as to distribute the weight of the leg along the calf without putting pressure on the Achilles tendon.[3,50–52] The knee should be in slight flexion.

TABLE 8.1	Overview of Support Surfaces
Low-tech devices	These provide a conforming support surface, distributing body weight over a large area. They include: • high-specification foam mattresses/overlays • air-filled mattresses/overlays
High-tech devices	These are dynamic systems and include: • alternating-pressure mattresses/overlays • air-fluidized beds/mattresses/overlays • low-air-loss overlays/mattresses/beds
Other devices	This group includes: • turning beds/frames (kinetic beds) • operating table overlays • (wheelchair) seat cushions • limb protectors

From McInnes E, Jammali-Blasi A, Bell-Syer SE, Dumville JC, Middleton V, Cullum N. Support surfaces for pressure ulcer prevention. *Cochrane Database Syst Rev*. 2015;(9):CD001735; Serraes B, van Leen M, Schols J, Van Hecke A, Verhaeghe S, Beeckman D. Prevention of pressure ulcers with a static air support surface: A systematic review. *Int Wound J*. 2018;15(3):333–343; and Vanderwee K, Grypdonck M, Defloor T. Alternating pressure air mattresses as prevention for pressure ulcers: a literature review. *Int J Nurs Stud*. 2008;45(5):784–801.

Patient repositioning is defined as changes of position in the lying or seated individual that aim to relieve or redistribute pressure and to enhance comfort. Repositioning at regular intervals is considered a cornerstone of PU prevention.[3] As a consequence, soft tissues and cells recover from sustained deformations, perfusion is restored and accumulated waste products eliminated, water evaporates, the stratum corneum hydration decreases and the skin surface temperature decreases.[53] According to the clinical practice guideline published in 2014,[3] repositioning and its frequency should take into account the condition of the individual and the applied support surface (e.g., pressure-relieving mattresses and cushions). Therefore, skin assessment and the observation of erythema is extremely important, as the presence of non-blanchable erythema plays a major role in developing individualized care plans.[3]

Previous research shows that different positions have an impact on tissue blood flow and interface pressure.[54,55] A study by Källman et al.[55] investigated six different lying positions (supine tilt 30°, supine 0°, semi-Fowler with elevated head 30°, semi-Fowler with elevated head and legs 30°, lateral 30° and lateral 90°) among 20 older hospitalized patients. The results showed that the median relative change in superficial blood flow over bony prominences increased in all supine positions and decreased in the lateral positions. The median relative change in the lateral 30° position was significantly lower than in all the supine positions. A lower median relative change of blood flow was also observed in the lateral 90° position in comparison with the supine tilt 30° position. The median relative change of blood flow over bony prominences in the deeper tissue increased in all positions.[55]

A study by Defloor[54] exploring the interface pressure in 10 different lying positions found that the 30° semi-Fowler position and the prone position resulted in the lowest interface pressure measurements. The lateral 30°

position had lower pressure readings, compared with the lateral 90° position which resulted in the highest interface pressure measurements.[54] Consequently, it is recommended to position patients lying in bed in the lateral 30° position, the prone position or the supine position.[3] Positions also have an impact when patients are seated in a chair. In a study by Giesbrecht et al.,[56] the relative reduction in interface pressure at the ischial tuberosities and the sacrum was measured with 10° increments of tilt in a manual wheelchair. The study revealed that a minimum tilt of 30° is needed to achieve a reduction in pressure.

DIFFERENTIAL DIAGNOSIS

Healthcare professionals often experience difficulties differentiating between PUs and IAD (Table 8.2).[40,57,58]

- Both skin injuries have different aetiologies but may co-exist.
- IAD is a 'top down' injury, while PUs are considered to be 'bottom up' injuries where damage is

TABLE 8.2 Differential Diagnosis: Pressure Ulcers and Incontinence-Associated Dermatitis

	Pressure Ulcers	Incontinence-Associated Dermatitis
History	Exposure to pressure and/or shear	Urinary and/or faecal incontinence
Location	Usually over a bony prominence or associated with location of a medical device	Affects perineum, perigenital area, buttocks, gluteal fold, medial and posterior aspects of upper thighs, lower back; IAD may occur over a bony prominence
Shape	Lesion is limited to one spot	Diffuse, different superficial spots are more likely to be IAD, may be blotchy or present as a kissing ulcer (copy lesion)
Edges	Distinct edges or margins	Diffuse or irregular edges
Depth	Varies from intact skin with non-blanchable erythema to full-thickness skin loss	Intact skin with erythema (blanchable or non-blanchable) with or without superficial, partial-thickness skin loss
Colour	If redness is non-blanchable, this is most likely a PU category I	Blanchable or non-blanchable erythema, pink or white surrounding skin due to maceration
Necrosis	A black necrotic scab on bony prominence is a PU category III or IV. If there is no or limited muscular mass underlying the necrosis, the lesion is a PU category IV	No necrosis

IAD, Incontinence-associated dermatitis; PU, pressure ulcer.
Adapted from Defloor T, Schoonhoven L, Fletcher J, et al. Statement of the European Pressure Ulcer Advisory Panel – pressure ulcer classification: differentiation between pressure ulcers and moisture lesions. *J Wound Ostomy Cont.* 2005;32(5):302-306; discussion 306; and Beeckman D, Schoonhoven L, Fletcher J, et al. Pressure ulcers and incontinence-associated dermatitis: effectiveness of the Pressure Ulcer Classification education tool on classification by nurses. *BMJ Qual Saf* 2010;19(5):e3.

initiated by changes within soft tissues below and within the skin.

- To aid correct differentiation between PUs and IAD, the PuClas educational e-learning tool[59] was developed based on the NPUAP/EPUAP International Pressure Ulcer Classification system.[3] The Skin Integrity Research Group (SKINT) at Ghent University developed the 4th Edition of PuClas. Access to PuClas4 is granted after online registration. (https://puclas4.ucvvgent.be/).[59]

Incontinence-Associated Dermatitis

INCONTINENCE AND IMPACT ON SKIN INTEGRITY

Incontinence is defined as 'any accidental or involuntary loss of urine from the bladder (urinary incontinence) or bowel motion, faeces or wind from the bowel (faecal incontinence)'.[60] Population studies from numerous countries have reported that urinary incontinence (UI) prevalence ranges between 5% and 70%, with most studies reporting a prevalence of any UI in the range of 25–45%.[61] Prevalence figures rise with increasing age, and in women aged over 70 years more than 40% of the population is affected by UI. Prevalence rates are higher in the 'elderly-elderly' and amongst nursing home patients.[62] The mean annual incidence of UI has been reported to range between 1% and 9%, while estimates of remission vary more, from 4% to 30%.[61] Faecal incontinence (FI) is a hidden problem, being under-diagnosed, under-investigated and under-treated. Up to 10% of adults can experience an episode of FI during their lifespan. The prevalence of FI in the adult population is estimated to be 0.8–6.2%. Recent research in North America showed a prevalence of 8.3% in adults living in the community.[63] Incontinence is one of the conditions whose long-term sufferers are most likely to encounter skin integrity issues.[64]

IAD: DEFINITION AND EPIDEMIOLOGY

Continuous exposure to urine and faeces is one of the most common causes of skin breakdown, commonly defined as IAD.[65] IAD is a specific type of irritant contact dermatitis characterized by erythema of the skin around the buttocks, perineum, gluteal cleft and other areas where friction and moisture (from incontinence) is present between skin, incontinence

materials, clothing and bed linen.[66] In the International Classification of Diseases 11th Revision (ICD-11), incontinence-related skin problems are coded as 'Diseases of the skin'; more specifically under the subcategory 'Irritant contact dermatitis due to friction, sweating or contact with body fluids' (https://icd.who.int/en). IAD is included in a broader group of skin conditions referred to as moisture-associated skin damage (MASD).[67] Traditionally, IAD has received little attention as a distinct skin disorder, and is regularly confused with category/stage I/II PU.[58,68]

Studies report prevalence figures of IAD between 5.6% and 50.0%, with incidence rates between 3.4% and 25.0%, depending on the type of clinical setting and population studied.[65] Most epidemiological studies are performed in small–sample, single–centre and long-term care settings.[64] A study of the prevalence of IAD among hospitalized acute care patients in the United States (n = 976) reported a prevalence of 27%.[69] A study using a large sample (n = 3713) of incontinent participants reported an overall IAD prevalence across different healthcare settings in two European countries of 6.1%.[70] Approximately one-third of people with faecal incontinence develop IAD.[71]

PATHOPHYSIOLOGY

IAD is caused by the continuous interplay between skin surface 'wetness', increased skin surface pH, digestive intestinal enzymes, repeated skin cleansing activities and an occlusive environment associated with diapers and incontinence pads.[72] Prolonged exposures to the above-mentioned irritants lead to stratum corneum (SC) damage. Excessive skin surface moisture leads to hyperhydration of the corneocytes and to disruption of the intercellular lipid bilayers. The corneocytes swell and the SC thickness increases.[65] Lipases and proteases attack the SC proteins and lipids.[66] An impaired skin barrier and occlusive skin conditions (e.g., caused by the use of diapers/incontinence pads) may further facilitate infiltration of the SC by *Candida albicans* and other irritants.[66] In addition, the recurrent use of water, skin cleansing agents and washcloths and towels leads to chemical and physical irritation of the skin (defined as friction). Limited mobility and limited ability to move independently cause additional friction and shear loads in the SC and the epidermis, diminishing the strength of the epidermal barrier further.[65]

CLINICAL PRESENTATION AND ASSESSMENT

The clinical presentation of IAD ranges from erythema (with or without loss of skin) to cutaneous infections (such as candidiasis). IAD is often associated with redness, rash or vesiculation. Although the lesions are superficial, they become slightly deeper when infected.[73] While IAD is a common complication, it remains underreported, neglected, and difficult to treat.[66] In 2018, SKINT at Ghent University, in collaboration with an international team of expert researchers and clinicians, published the Ghent Global IAD Categorisation tool (GLOBIAD) (Box 8.3).[74] The tool was the result of a 2-year project involving 22 international experts and 823 clinicians from 30 countries. GLOBIAD categorizes IAD severity based on visual inspection of the affected skin areas. The purpose of the tool was to create an internationally agreed description of IAD severity, and to standardize the documentation of this condition in clinical practice and research.[73] The tool is now implemented in many countries.

RISK

Although the presence of incontinence is a prerequisite, not all incontinent patients develop IAD.[65] This indicates that many more factors and characteristics increase (i.e., act as a risk factor) or decrease (i.e., act as a protecting factor) the individual susceptibility or risk for IAD development. Many factors influence an individual's likelihood of developing IAD and effective prevention focuses on reducing the risk factors and strengthening the protective factors that are most closely related to IAD development. A risk factor is any attribute, characteristic or exposure of an individual that increases the likelihood of developing a disease or injury.[75] They are associated with a higher likelihood of negative outcomes. Protective factors are characteristics associated with a lower likelihood of negative outcomes or that reduce the impact of the risk factor. Protective factors may be considered as positive countering events.

Risk prediction models that typically use a number of patient characteristics to predict health outcomes are a cornerstone of modern clinical medicine and guide decision making. Despite research into IAD risk factors and prognostic models, this area is in its infancy. Merely based on expert opinion and cross-sectional studies, the following predictors are considered to increase IAD risk: constantly moist skin, age-related skin damage, type of incontinence, increased body mass index, presence of diabetes mellitus, friction and shear problems during patient movement.[65,76,77] In practice, IAD datasets used in risk model development often contain few events compared with the number of potential predictors.

PREVENTION AND MANAGEMENT

A 2016 Cochrane systematic review[64] concluded that little evidence exists on the effects of interventions for preventing and treating IAD in adults, and it is of very low to moderate quality. Soap and water performed poorly in the prevention and treatment of IAD. The application of leave-on products (moisturizers, skin protectants or a combination) and avoiding soap seems to be more effective than withholding these products. The performance of leave-on products depends on the combination of ingredients, the overall formulation and the usage (e.g., amount applied). High-quality confirmatory trials using standardized and comparable prevention and treatment regimens in different settings/regions are required. To increase the comparability of trial results, the development of an agreed minimum set of outcome domains and outcome measurement instruments that should be reported in all IAD trials was recommended.[64] A study published in 2018 using erythema, erosion, maceration, IAD-related pain and patient satisfaction as the five core outcomes to be measured and reported was undertaken.[78] No work has been done to systematically search for psychometrically valid and reliable measurement instruments for IAD-related erosion, maceration, pain and patient satisfaction so far.

BOX 8.3 THE GHENT GLOBAL IAD CATEGORISATION TOOL (GLOBIAD)

CATEGORY 1A: PERSISTENT REDNESS WITHOUT CLINICAL SIGNS OF INFECTION

Critical Criterion

- Persistent redness. A variety of tones of redness may be present. In patients with darker skin tones, the skin may be paler or darker than normal, or purple in colour.

Additional Criteria

- Marked areas or discolouration from a previous (healed) skin defect.
- Shiny appearance of the skin.
- Macerated skin.
- Intact vesicles and/or bullae.
- Skin may feel tense or swollen at palpation.
- Burning, tingling, itching or pain.

CATEGORY 1B: PERSISTENT REDNESS WITH CLINICAL SIGNS OF INFECTION

Critical Criteria

- Persistent redness. A variety of tones of redness may be present. In patients with darker skin tones, the skin may be paler or darker than normal, or purple in colour.
- Signs of infection, such as white scaling of the skin (suggesting a fungal infection) or satellite lesions (pustules surrounding the lesion, suggesting a *Candida albicans* fungal infection).

Additional Criteria

- Marked areas or discolouration from a previous (healed) skin defect.
- Shiny appearance of the skin.
- Macerated skin.
- Intact vesicles and/or bullae.
- Skin may feel tense or swollen at palpation.
- Burning, tingling, itching or pain.

CATEGORY 2A: SKIN LOSS WITHOUT CLINICAL SIGNS OF INFECTION

Critical Criterion

- Skin loss may present as skin erosion (may result from damaged/eroded vesicles or bullae), denudation or excoriation. The skin damage pattern may be diffuse.

Additional Criteria

- Persistent redness. A variety of tones of redness may be present. In patients with darker skin tones, the skin may be paler or darker than normal, or purple in colour.
- Marked areas or discolouration from a previous (healed) skin defect.
- Shiny appearance of the skin.
- Macerated skin.
- Intact vesicles and/or bullae.
- Skin may feel tense or swollen at palpation.
- Burning, tingling, itching or pain.

CATEGORY 2B: SKIN LOSS WITH CLINICAL SIGNS OF INFECTION

Critical Criteria

- Skin loss may present as skin erosion (may result from damaged/eroded vesicles or bullae), denudation or excoriation. The skin damage pattern may be diffuse.
- Signs of infection, such as white scaling of the skin (suggesting a fungal infection) or satellite lesions (pustules surrounding the lesion, suggesting a *Candida albicans* fungal infection), slough visible in the wound bed (yellow/brown/greyish), green appearance within the wound bed (suggesting a bacterial infection with *Pseudomonas aeruginosa*), excessive exudate levels, purulent exudate (pus) or a shiny appearance of the wound bed.

Additional Criteria

Persistent redness. A variety of tones of redness may be present. In patients with darker skin tones, the skin may be paler or darker than normal, or purple in colour.

Marked areas or discolouration from a previous (healed) skin defect.

Shiny appearance of the skin.

Macerated skin.

Intact vesicles and/or bullae.

Skin may feel tense or swollen at palpation.

Burning, tingling, itching or pain.

Reproduced with permission from Beeckman D, Van den Bussche K, Alves P, et al. The Ghent Global IAD Categorisation. Skin Integrity Research Group: Ghent University; 2017. Available from: https://www.skintghent.be/en

REFERENCES

1. United Nations. *World Population Ageing*; 2015. Available from: http://www.un.org/en/development/desa/population/theme/ageing/WPA2015.shtml.
2. Hahnel E, Lichterfeld A, Blume-Peytavi U, Kottner J. The epidemiology of skin conditions in the aged: a systematic review. *J Tissue Viability*. 2017;26(1):20–28.
3. National pressure ulcer Advisory Panel (US), European pressure ulcer Advisory Panel, Pan Pacific pressure injury Alliance. In: Haesler E, ed. *Prevention and Treatment of Pressure Ulcers: A Clinical Practice Guideline*. Osborne Park, Australia: Cambridge Media; 2014.
4. Vanderwee K, Defloor T, Beeckman D, et al. Assessing the adequacy of pressure ulcer prevention in hospitals: a nationwide prevalence survey. *BMJ Qual Saf*. 2011;20(3):260 267.
5. Demarré L, Verhaeghe S, Annemans L, Van Hecke A, Grypdonck M, Beeckman D. The cost of pressure ulcer prevention and treatment in hospitals and nursing homes in flanders: a cost-of-illness study. *Int J Nurs Stud*. 2015;52(7):1166–1179.
6. Demarré L, Van Lancker A, Van Hecke A, et al. The cost of pre-

vention and treatment of pressure ulcers: a systematic review. *Int J Nurs Stud.* 2015;52(11):1754–1774.

7. Hopkins A, Dealey C, Bale S, Defloor T, Worboys F. Patient stories of living with a pressure ulcer. *J Adv Nurs.* 2006;56(4):345–353.

8. Gorecki C, Brown JM, Nelson EA, et al. Impact of pressure ulcers on quality of life in older patients: a systematic review. *J Am Geriatr Soc.* 2009;57(7):1175–1183.

9. Essex HN, Clark M, Sims J, Warriner A, Cullum N. Health-related quality of life in hospital inpatients with pressure ulceration: assessment using generic health-related quality of life measures. *Wound Repair Regen.* 2009;17(6):797–805.

10. Coleman S, Nixon J, Keen J, et al. A new pressure ulcer conceptual framework. *J Adv Nurs.* 2014;70(10):2222–2234.

11. Breuls RGM, Bouten CVC, Oomens CWJ, Bader DL, Baaijens FPT. Compression induced cell damage in engineered muscle tissue: an in vitro model to study pressure ulcer aetiology. *Ann Biomed Eng.* 2003;31(11):1357–1364.

12. Breuls RG, Bouten CV, Oomens CW, Bader DL, Baaijens FP. A theoretical analysis of damage evolution in skeletal muscle tissue with reference to pressure ulcer development. *J Biomech Eng.* 2003;125(6):902–909.

13. Gawlitta D, Li W, Oomens CWJ, Baaijens FPT, Bader DL, Bouten CVC. The relative contributions of compression and hypoxia to development of muscle tissue damage: an in vitro study. *Ann Biomed Eng.* 2007;35(2):273–284.

14. Gawlitta D, Oomens CWJ, Bader DL, Baaijens FPT, Bouten CVC. Temporal differences in the influence of ischemic factors and deformation on the metabolism of engineered skeletal muscle. *J Appl Physiol.* 2007;103(2):464–473.

15. Linder-Ganz E, Engelberg S, Scheinowitz M, Gefen A. Pressure-time cell death threshold for albino rat skeletal muscles as related to pressure sore biomechanics. *J Biomech.* 2006;39(14):2725–2732.

16. Salcido R, Donofrio JC, Fisher SB, et al. Histopathology of pressure ulcers as a result of sequential computer-controlled pressure sessions in a fuzzy rat model. *Adv Wound Care.* 1994;7(5):23–4, 26, 28 passim.

17. Stekelenburg A, Oomens CWJ, Strijkers GJ, Nicolay K, Bader DL. Compression-induced deep tissue injury examined with magnetic resonance imaging and histology. *J Appl Physiol.* 2006;100(6):1946–1954.

18. Wounds International. *International Review. Pressure Ulcer Prevention Pressure Shear Friction and Microclimate in Context. A Consensus Document;* 2010. Available from: https://www .woundsinternational.com/resources/details/international-review-pressure-ulcer-prevention-pressure-shear-friction-and-microclimate-context.

19. Bader DL, Barnhill RL, Ryan TJ. Effect of externally applied skin surface forces on tissue vasculature. *Arch Phys Med Rehabil.* 1986;67(11):807–811.

20. Dinsdale SM. Decubitus ulcers: role of pressure and friction in causation. *Arch Phys Med Rehabil.* 1974;55(4):147–152.

21. Kosiak M. Etiology of decubitus ulcers. *Arch Phys Med Rehabil.* 1961;42:19–29.

22. Berecek KH. Etiology of decubitus ulcers. *Nurs Clin North Am.* 1975;10(1):157–170.

23. Berlowitz DR, Brienza DM. Are all pressure ulcers the result of deep tissue injury? A review of the literature. *Ostomy Wound Manage.* 2007;53(10):34–38.

24. Daniel RK, Priest DL, Wheatley DC. Etiologic factors in pressure sores: an experimental model. *Arch Phys Med Rehabil.*

1981;62(10):492–498.

25. Edsberg LE. Pressure ulcer tissue histology: an appraisal of current knowledge. *Ostomy Wound Manage.* 2007;53(10):40–49.

26. Nola GT, Vistnes LM. Differential response of skin and muscle in the experimental production of pressure sores. *Plast Reconstr Surg.* 1980;66(5):728–733.

27. Loerakker S, Manders E, Strijkers GJ, et al. The effects of deformation, ischemia, and reperfusion on the development of muscle damage during prolonged loading. *J Appl Physiol.* 2011;111(4):1168–1177.

28. Loerakker S, Oomens CWJ, Manders E, et al. Ischemia-reperfusion injury in rat skeletal muscle assessed with T2-weighted and dynamic contrast-enhanced MRI. *Magn Reson Med.* 2011;66(2):528–537.

29. Houwing R, Overgoor M, Kon M, Jansen G, van Asbeck BS, Haalboom JRE. Pressure-induced skin lesions in pigs: reperfusion injury and the effects of vitamin E. *J Wound Care.* 2000;9(1):36–40.

30. Ikebe M, Komatsu S, Woodhead JL, et al. The tip of the coiled-coil rod determines the filament formation of smooth muscle and nonmuscle myosin. *J Biol Chem.* 2001;276(32):30293–30300.

31. Peirce SM, Skalak TC, Rodeheaver GT. Ischemia-reperfusion injury in chronic pressure ulcer formation: a skin model in the rat. *Wound Repair Regen.* 2019;8(1):68–76.

32. Reid RR, Sull AC, Mogford JE, Roy N, Mustoe TA. A novel murine model of cyclical cutaneous ischemia-reperfusion injury. *J Surg Res.* 2004;116(1):172–180.

33. Tsuji S, Ichioka S, Sekiya N, Nakatsuka T. Analysis of ischemia-reperfusion injury in a microcirculatory model of pressure ulcers. *Wound Repair Regen.* 2005;13(2):209–215.

34. Unal S, Ozmen S, Demir Y, et al. The effect of gradually increased blood flow on ischemia-reperfusion injury. *Ann Plast Surg.* 2001;47(4):412–416.

35. Ceelen KK, Stekelenburg A, Loerakker S, et al. Compression-induced damage and internal tissue strains are related. *J Biomech.* 2008;41(16):3399–3404.

36. Stekelenburg A, Gawlitta D, Bader DL, Oomens CW. Deep tissue injury: how deep is our understanding? *Arch Phys Med Rehabil.* 2008;89(7):1410–1413.

37. Stekelenburg A, Strijkers GJ, Parusel H, Bader DL, Nicolay K, Oomens CW. Role of ischemia and deformation in the onset of compression-induced deep tissue injury: MRI-based studies in a rat model. *J Appl Physiol.* 2007;102(5):2002–2011.

38. Loerakker S, Stekelenburg A, Strijkers GJ, et al. Temporal effects of mechanical loading on deformation-induced damage in skeletal muscle tissue. *Ann Biomed Eng.* 2010;38(8):2577–2587.

39. Bouten CV, Oomens CW, Baaijens FP, Bader DL. The etiology of pressure ulcers: skin deep or muscle bound? *Arch Phys Med Rehabil.* 2003;84(4):616–619.

40. Defloor T, Schoonhoven L. Inter-rater reliability of the EPUAP pressure ulcer classification system using photographs. *J Clin Nurs.* 2004;13(8):952–959.

41. Nixon J, Thorpe H, Barrow H, et al. Reliability of pressure ulcer classification and diagnosis. *J Adv Nurs.* 2005;50(6):613–623.

42. Schuurman J-P, Schoonhoven L, Defloor T, van Engelshoven I, van Ramshorst B, Buskens E. Economic evaluation of pressure ulcer care: a cost minimization analysis of preventive strategies. *Nurs Econ.* 2009;27(6):390–400, 415.

43. *NICE. Pressure Ulcers: Prevention and Management Guidance and Guidelines NICE.* National Institute for Health and Care Excellence;

2014. Available from: https://www.nice.org.uk/guidance/cg179.

44. Defloor T, Bacquer DD, Grypdonck MHF. The effect of various combinations of turning and pressure reducing devices on the incidence of pressure ulcers. *Int J Nurs Stud.* 2005;42(1):37–46.

45. National Pressure Ulcer Advisory Panel. Terms and definitions related to support surfaces; 2007. Available from: https://npuap.org/page/S3I.

46. McInnes E, Jammali-Blasi A, Bell-Syer SE, Dumville JC, Middleton V, Cullum N. Support surfaces for pressure ulcer prevention. *Cochrane Database Syst Rev.* 2015;9:CD001735.

47. Shi C, Dumville JC, Cullum N. Support surfaces for pressure ulcer prevention: a network meta-analysis. *PLoS One.* 2018;13(2):e0192707.

48. Serraes B, van Leen M, Schols J, Van Hecke A, Verhaeghe S, Beeckman D. Prevention of pressure ulcers with a static air support surface: a systematic review. *Int Wound J.* 2018;15(3):333–343.

49. Vanderwee K, Grypdonck M, Defloor T. Alternating pressure air mattresses as prevention for pressure ulcers: a literature review. *Int J Nurs Stud.* 2008;45(5):784–801.

50. Donnelly J. Hospital-acquired heel ulcers: a common but neglected problem. *J Wound Care.* 2001;10(4):131–136.

51. Heyneman A, Vanderwee K, Grypdonck M, Defloor T. Effectiveness of two cushions in the prevention of heel pressure ulcers. *Worldviews Evidence-Based Nurs.* 2009;6(2):114–120.

52. Wong VK, Stotts NA. Physiology and prevention of heel ulcers: the state of science. *J Wound Ostomy Cont.* 2003;30(4):191–198.

53. Worsley PR, Parsons B, Bader DL. An evaluation of fluid immersion therapy for the prevention of pressure ulcers. *Clin Biomech.* 2016;40:27–32.

54. Defloor T. The effect of position and mattress on interface pressure. *Appl Nurs Res.* 2000;1:2–11.

55. Källman U, Bergstrand S, Ek A-C, Engström M, Lindberg L-G, Lindgren M. Different lying positions and their effects on tissue blood flow and skin temperature in older adult patients. *J Adv Nurs.* 2013;69(1):133–144.

56. Giesbrecht EM, Ethans KD, Staley D. Measuring the effect of incremental angles of wheelchair tilt on interface pressure among individuals with spinal cord injury. *Spinal Cord.* 2011;49(7):827–831.

57. Defloor T, Schoonhoven L, Fletcher J, et al. Statement of the European Pressure Ulcer Advisory Panel–pressure ulcer classification: differentiation between pressure ulcers and moisture lesions. *J Wound Ostomy Cont.* 2019;32(5):302–306; discussion 306.

58. Beeckman D, Schoonhoven L, Fletcher J, et al. Pressure ulcers and incontinence-associated dermatitis: effectiveness of the Pressure Ulcer Classification education tool on classification by nurses. *BMJ Qual Saf.* 2010;19(5):e3.

59. Beeckman D. *European Pressure Ulcer Advisory Panel. PuClas4 eLearning Module.* University Centre for Nursing & Midwifery and European Pressure Ulcer Advisory Pane; 2017. Available from: https://puclas4.ucvvgent.be/.

60. Abrams P, Cardozo L, Wagg A, Wein AJ, Alan J. *International Continence Society.* Tokyo: Incontinence: 6th International Consultation on Incontinence; 2016:2519. Available from: https://www.ics.org/education/icspublications/icibooks/6thicibook.

61. Milsom I, Gyhagen M. The prevalence of urinary incontinence. *Climacteric.* 2019;22(3):217–222.

62. Hunskaar S, Lose G, Sykes D, Voss S. The prevalence of urinary incontinence in women in four European countries. *BJU Int.* 2004;93(3):324–330.

63. Nazarko L. Faecal incontinence: investigation, treatment and management. *Br J Community Nurs.* 2018;23(12):582–588.

64. Beeckman D, Van Damme N, Schoonhoven L, et al. Interventions for preventing and treating incontinence-associated dermatitis in adults. *Cochrane Database Syst Rev.* 2016;11:CD011627.

65. Kottner J, Beeckman D. Incontinence-associated dermatitis and pressure ulcers in geriatric patients. *G Ital Dermatol Venereol.* 2015;150(6):717–729.

66. Gray M, Beeckman D, Bliss DZ, et al. Incontinence-associated dermatitis: a comprehensive review and update. *J Wound Ostomy Cont.* 2012;39(1):61–74.

67. Woo KY, Beeckman D, Chakravarthy D. Management of moisture-associated skin damage: a Scoping review. *Adv Skin Wound Care.* 2017,30(11):494–501.

68. Beeckman D, Van Lancker A, Van Hecke A, Verhaeghe S. A systematic review and meta-analysis of incontinence-associated dermatitis, incontinence, and moisture as risk factors for pressure ulcer development. *Res Nurs Health.* 2014;37(3):204–218.

69. Gray M, Giuliano KK. Incontinence-associated dermatitis, characteristics and relationship to pressure injury: a multisite epidemiologic analysis. *J Wound Ostomy Cont.* 2017;45(1):63–67.

70. Kottner J, Blume-Peytavi U, Lohrmann C, Halfens R. Associations between individual characteristics and incontinence-associated dermatitis: a secondary data analysis of a multi-centre prevalence study. *Int J Nurs Stud.* 2014;51(10):1373–1380.

71. Doughty D, Junkin J, Kurz P, et al. Incontinence-associated dermatitis: consensus statements, evidence-based guidelines for prevention and treatment, and current challenges. *J Wound Ostomy Cont.* 2012;39(3):303–315.

72. Beele H, Smet S, Van Damme N, Beeckman D. Incontinence-associated dermatitis: pathogenesis, contributing factors, prevention and management options. *Drugs Aging.* 2018;35(1):1–10.

73. Beeckman D, Van den Bussche K, Alves P, et al. Towards an international language for incontinence-associated dermatitis (IAD): design and evaluation of psychometric properties of the Ghent Global IAD Categorization Tool (GLOBIAD) in 30 countries. *Br J Dermatol.* 2018;178(6):1331–1340.

74. Beeckman D, Van den Bussche K, Alves P, et al. *The Ghent Global IAD Categorisation. Skin Integrity Research Group.* Ghent University; 2017. Available from: https://www.skintghent.be/en/onderzoek/Tools/2/incontinence-associated-dermatitis-iad.

75. Coleman S, Smith IL, McGinnis E, et al. Clinical evaluation of a new pressure ulcer risk assessment instrument, the pressure ulcer risk primary or secondary evaluation tool (PURPOSE T). *J Adv Nurs.* 2018;74(2):407–424.

76. Van Damme N, Van den Bussche K, De Meyer D, Van Hecke A, Verhaeghe S, Beeckman D. Independent risk factors for the development of skin erosion due to incontinence (incontinence-associated dermatitis category 2) in nursing home residents: results from a multivariate binary regression analysis. *Int Wound J.* 2017;14(5):801–810.

77. Van Damme N, Clays E, Verhaeghe S, Van Hecke A, Beeckman D. Independent risk factors for the development of incontinence-associated dermatitis (category 2) in critically ill patients with fecal incontinence: a cross-sectional observational study in 48 ICU units. *Int J Nurs Stud.* 2018;81:30–39.

78. Van den Bussche K, Kottner J, Beele H, et al. Core outcome domains in incontinence-associated dermatitis research. *J Adv Nurs.* 2018;74(7):1605–1617.

    Manderlier B, Van Damme N, Vanderwee K, Verhaeghe S, Van Hecke A, Beeckman D. Development and psychometric validation of PUKAT 2·0, a knowledge assessment tool for pressure ulcer prevention. *Int Wound J.* 2017;14(6):1041–1051.

MCQS

1   *A patient sits with the head of the bed elevated to 60°. What happens when his skin sticks to the underlying surface while he slides down in the bed?*
   a. The pressure increases
   b. Problems with the microclimate occur (temperature and relative humidity)
   c. Shear increases
   d. Friction/rubbing increases

2   *In which of these categories can necrotic tissue be present?*
   a. Category I, II, III and IV
   b. Category II, III and IV
   c. Category III and IV
   d. Category IV only

3   *Which repositioning protocol is most effective to prevent PUs? Starting with the patient supine, then:*
   a. Lateral 30° left – supine – lateral 30° right – supine – lateral 30° left …
   b. Lateral 90° left – supine – lateral 90° right – supine – lateral 90° left …
   c. Lateral 30° left – supine – lateral 30° right – supine – lateral 90° left – supine – lateral 90° right …
   d. Lateral 30° left – lateral 90° left – supine –lateral 30° right – lateral 90° right – supine …

Chapter 9

Wound Care in Elderly Individuals with Leg Ulcerations

Paul Bobbink

Highlights

As you go through this chapter, pay attention to the following:

- The importance of correctly assessing leg ulceration
- The importance of understanding the basic principles of leg ulcer management
- The importance of the nurse–patient relationship (during treatment) in supporting patients living with their wounds

Key Issues

This chapter focuses on leg ulcerations with various aetiologies (venous, arterial or mixed), which are common in the elderly population.

Clinical Case Studies

Aetiology and management of:

- A woman suffering from a venous ulceration
- A man suffering from a mixed leg ulceration

Introduction

The general challenges in wound management in elderly patients were discussed in the introduction to Chapter 8. This chapter focuses on the management of leg ulcerations (LUs) with various aetiologies. First, the epidemiological data and background of LUs will be presented. Then, the chapter will focus on global and specific LU management depending on the wound's aetiology.

Definition, Epidemiology and Consequences

An LU is defined as a loss of skin on the lower leg or foot that takes more than 6 weeks to heal.[1] In industrialized countries, the prevalence of leg ulcerations in the general population is about 0.5–1% and increases with age. In the population over 80 years of age, the the prevalence rise up to 3%.[2–4] These numbers are constantly increasing and show that leg ulcers are common in the elderly.[3,4]

The healthcare cost associated with LU treatment in the UK is estimated at £1.94 billion per year.[5] In Germany, the mean estimated cost increased to €9060 per patient per year.[6] Reviewing the use of healthcare resources for wound care, it is clear that the management of LUs falls predominantly to community nurses.[5,7]

Some socio-demographic factors can be associated with LUs. Moffat et al.[8] states that LUs are predominant in lower social classes and in individuals living alone.

Generally, LUs take a long time – sometimes years – to heal. In the specific case of venous leg ulcers, 60% will heal within 6 months, 33% in 1 year and 7% will never heal.[9] Once healed, they present a high recurrence rate, estimated at 69% in 1 year.[2]

The impact on daily life for patients with LUs is well documented.[10] The most commonly experienced symptoms are pain, immobility, insomnia, exudate and odour.[10] Anxiety, depression and social life restriction are also well documented consequences.[11] Edwards and colleagues[12] showed that 64% of patients with LUs suffer from four or more symptoms. Additionally, outdoor mobility and finding appropriate footwear are also important problems for patients.[13]

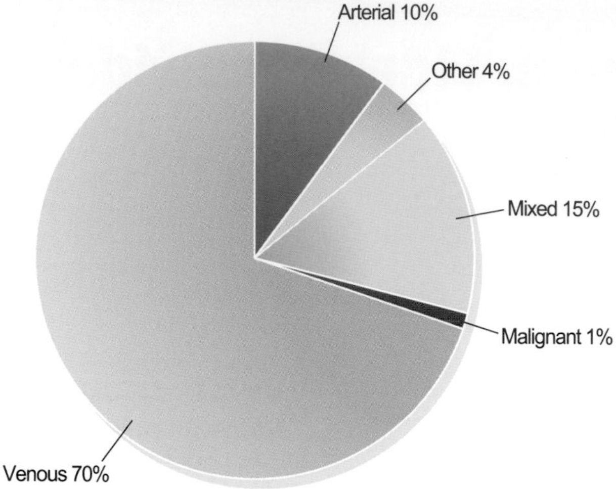

Arterial 10%

Other 4%

Mixed 15%

Malignant 1%

Venous 70%

Fig. 9.1 Aetiology of leg ulcers.

LUs are generally a symptom of vascular disease. They can originate from various aetiologies, such as venous, arterial or mixed. The aetiologies are shown in Fig. 9.1.

Aetiology

VENOUS AETIOLOGY

The venous system of the lower leg pumps blood back towards the heart. As this action takes place against gravity in the human, this is difficult to achieve.

There are three categories of vein within the legs: deep, superficial and communicating (perforator) veins. The superficial long and short saphenous veins (draining the skin) pump blood under low pressure into the deep venous system through the perforators (Fig. 9.2). The deep veins are surrounded by muscles (the calf muscle pump) which contract and relax during walking to pump blood up the leg. Healthy venous return is achieved not only by walking (so using the calf muscle pump) but also by having full ankle movement; when the ankle moves, the Achilles tendon contracts and releases, to assist the calf muscle pump.

Damage to the venous system can occur at any time of life. Deep vein thrombosis and varicose veins damage the perforators, making them incompetent (Fig. 9.3). Immobility of and arthritic changes to the

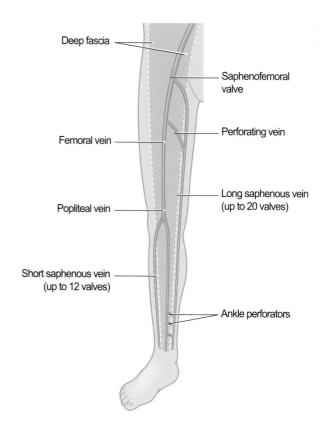

Deep fascia

Saphenofemoral valve

Perforating vein

Femoral vein

Long saphenous vein (up to 20 valves)

Popliteal vein

Short saphenous vein (up to 12 valves)

Ankle perforators

Fig. 9.2 The normal venous system of the leg.

ankle joint impair ankle movement and so further impede venous return.

Failure of the calf muscle pump results in backflow of blood and pooling, causing venous hypertension, which leads to oedema of the lower leg and pigmentation of the 'gaiter' area.[14] This pigmentation is the result of haemoglobin being released from red blood cells which have leaked out of the distended blood capillaries and deposited haemosiderin. Also, the subsequent rise in ambulatory pressure is believed to enlarge and increase the permeability of the local capillary bed, allowing molecules such as fibrinogen to escape into the interstitial fluid. Fibrinogen is then formed into insoluble fibrin complexes, which form a cuff around capillaries, affecting oxygen diffusion into the tissues. This so-called 'fibrin cuff theory' was first proposed by Burnand et al.[15] The gradual replacement of skin and subcutaneous tissue by fibrous tissue also explains the appearance of 'woody skin', a condition called lipodermatosclerosis, commonly seen in patients with venous ulceration.[16]

Other explanations for causation have been given, mostly related to the 'white cell trapping' theory,[17] where it is believed that following an episode of deep vein thrombosis or phlebitis, white cells increase and become trapped in the capillaries of the leg. Here they release toxic substances such as oxygen free radicals, causing tissue death. This underlying problem is soon revealed when a subsequent knock or minor injury to this area of the lower leg rapidly leads to ulceration. Venous leg ulcerations (VLUs) most commonly occur around the gaiter area (Fig. 9.4) where usually the ulcers are shallow.

ARTERIAL AETIOLOGY

The heart pumps blood to the organs and to the extremities via the arterial system (Fig. 9.5A). Reduction of arterial flow, as occurs in a progressive disease like atherosclerosis or due to an acute thrombotic event, causes tissue ischemia and can lead to an arterial leg ulcer (ALU). Patients may complain of intermittent claudication (pain on walking), ischaemic rest pain (pain often coming on at night when in bed) or episodes of critical limb ischaemia (requires prompt vascular attention). The condition will usually be

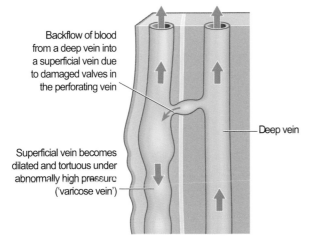

Backflow of blood from a deep vein into a superficial vein due to damaged valves in the perforating vein

Deep vein

Superficial vein becomes dilated and tortuous under abnormally high pressure ('varicose vein')

Fig. 9.3 A damaged venous system: an incompetent valve in a perforating vein allows backflow of blood from the deep to the superficial venous system.

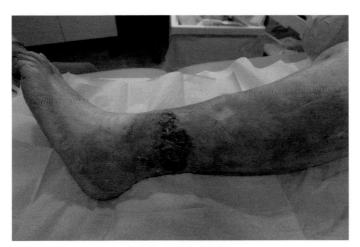

Fig. 9.4 A venous leg ulcer.

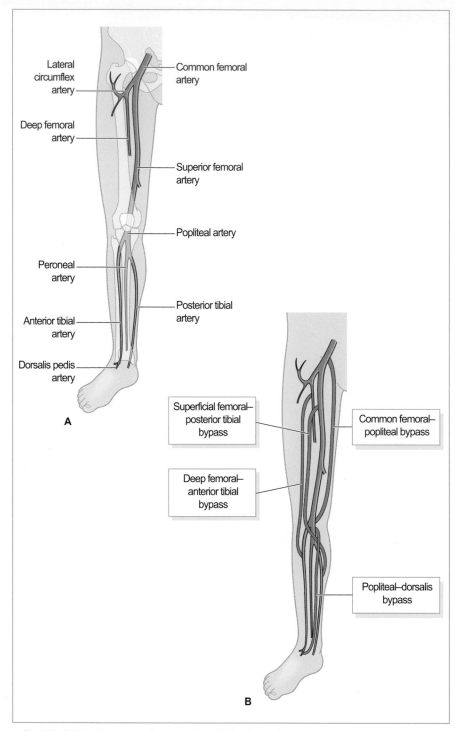

Lateral circumflex artery

Common femoral artery

Deep femoral artery

Superior femoral artery

Popliteal artery

Peroneal artery

Posterior tibial artery

Anterior tibial artery

Dorsalis pedis artery

A

Superficial femoral–posterior tibial bypass

Common femoral–popliteal bypass

Deep femoral–anterior tibial bypass

Popliteal–dorsalis bypass

B

Fig. 9.5 (A) Arterial anatomy of a normal limb. (B) Surgical options for revascularizing the lower limb.

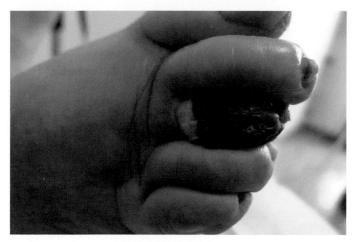

Fig. 9.6 An arterial leg ulcer.

accompanied by other circulatory disorders such as hypertension, cerebral vascular accidents and myocardial infarctions. One-third of patients who present with ulceration will have critical limb ischaemia.[18]

Arterial ulcers are usually found on the distal parts of the digits, over bony prominences and on the dorsum of the foot (Fig. 9.6).

Skin in the Elderly

Skin changes with age. The thinning of the epidermis, loss of collagen and decreased activity of sebaceous glands are factors that make the skin more fragile and place it at risk of skin tears.[19] For further details, Blume-Peytavi et al. provide a helpful overview.[20]

Assessment of a Person with an Ulcerated Leg

The assessment of the patient requires a holistic approach, taking into account the experience of living with an LU and a physical assessment that includes the LU itself. The structure and content of data collection will be influenced by the nursing model or theory used. However, if we focus on wound care in nursing, some elements have to be taken into consideration for effective LU management. The patient's comprehensive medical history helps determine the wound's aetiology (Table 9.1). Furthermore, symptom evaluation and clarification of the consequences of living with an

LU are important because they will affect LU management and the patient's adherence to wound care.[21,22]

Fig. 9.7 illustrates the specific assessment for a holistic approach to LU management.

Green et al.[23] observed that patients did not always mention their concerns to the nurse during the consultation. However, when they did, nurses often overlooked, ignored or did not manage the patient's concerns. In fact, Heinen et al.[13] stated that patients did not receive care related to problems caused by the LU. The main unaddressed problems were sleep (73%) and negative effects of compression (71%) or footwear (70%). The data demonstrates the complex and multifaceted nature of the nurse–patient relationship during LU treatment.

Some research tools could help nurses better assess patients' needs during treatment. Augustin et al.[24] developed a tool to assess patients' specific needs while they suffered from chronic wounds. Some of the questions are presented in Box 9.1 and can easily be adapted for everyday use in clinical practice.

PAIN AND SYMPTOM ASSESSMENT

Pain is frequently present with LUs, but the form and description of pain differs in arterial and venous LUs. In VLUs, pain will be described as aching, and in ALUs, it will be described as cramps, which increase with exercise.[25] Leg pain is intensified in VLUs after the patient sits for a long time, whereas this position may be pain-relieving in ALUs. In ALUs, pain also indicates arterial disease. First, pain will be present when the

TABLE 9.1	A Global Assessment Orientated Toward Aetiology		
	Venous Aetiology	**Arterial Aetiology**	**Mixed Aetiology**
Medical history	Advanced age Deep vein thrombosis Leg injury History of phlebitis	Cardiac disease Hypertension Stroke Renal disease Smoking history	Smoking history Cardiac disease Hypertension Stroke Renal disease
Leg assessment	'Heavy leg' Varicose veins Lipodermatosclerosis Atrophie blanche and/or skin pigmentation Oedema	Pale leg Leg hair reduction Non-palpable distal pulse Thin skin	Clinical signs of VLU and ALU A non-palpable pulse, pale and hairless leg, thin skin could orient to MLU
Peripheral skin assessment	Stasis eczema Contact dermatitis	Cool, pale and dry skin	Both elements could be present depending on the gravity of each disease
Wound bed assessment	Superficial wound Rarely extends to tendons or bones Exudative Slough/fibrinous Localized around the malleolus	Deep wound Bones or tendons could be exposed Dry Necrotic Localized on toe, outside of the foot or bony prominences	At first impression looks like a VLU but: Wound is often "deeper" than VLU with more devitalized tissue

patient walks and after disease progression when the patient lies flat in bed, which is called 'rest pain'.

Physical Assessment

The literature shows that patients need a clear diagnosis and therapy.[24,26] From a medical point of view, effective management of an LU also requires an accurate diagnosis of its aetiology.[27] Therefore, it is crucial that nurses can effectively assess a wound's aetiology.

The causation of an LU is primarily confirmed by physical examination. In an assessment of both legs, the skin reaching to the extremities must be inspected. The objective data will likely confirm the patient's medical history and the signs and symptoms expressed by the patient.

During an assessment, nurses may identify clinical symptoms, such as oedema, varicose veins or varicosities, which indicate venous disease (Fig. 9.8). The clinical – (a)etiology – anatomy – pathophysiology (CEAP) (Table 9.2) classification provides more information about the gravity of the venous disease.[28] Inversely, intermittent claudication, a low-temperature foot or leg or a pale toe indicates arterial disease. The Fontaine classification gives more information

about the gravity of the peripheral arterial disease (PAD; Table 9.3).[29] This assessment must be carefully performed because 15–25% of LUs have a coexisting arteriovenous disease.[27,30] The clinical differences for leg assessment are summarized in Table 9.1.

The mixed leg ulcer (MLU) presents characteristics of venous and arterial dysfunction. A descriptive study from 2017 showed that an MLU was associated with hairless, shiny, taut and cracked skin in comparison with a VLU.[30] Any suspicion of either aetiology must be clarified.

During examination, further investigations can be performed. For example, the ankle–brachial pressure index (ABPI; also called the ankle–brachial index – ABI) is defined as the ratio between the arm and ankle systolic blood pressure. ABPI is a non-invasive method that permits the identification of PAD also, in case of the leg, called lower extremity artery disease (LEAD).

The ABPI is calculated as:

$$\frac{\text{ankle systolic pressure}}{\text{brachial systolic pressure}} = \text{ankle brachial pressure index}$$

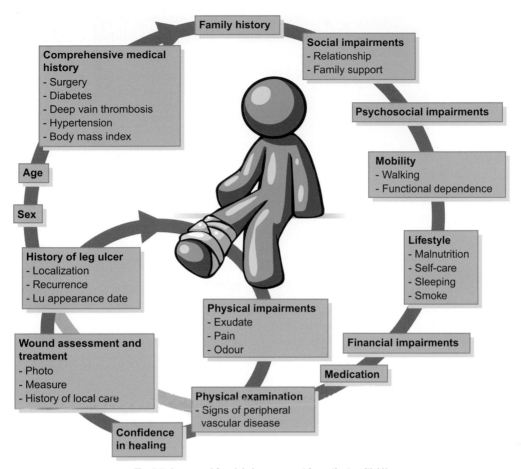

Fig. 9.7 A proposal for global assessment for patients with LU.

BOX 9.1 ASSESSING PATIENTS' NEEDS

How important is it for you to:
- be able to lead a normal everyday life
- be able to engage in normal leisure activities
- be less burdened in partnership
- not have an unpleasant smell from the lesion
- have fewer side effects
- be able to sleep better
- be less dependent on doctor and clinic visits
- need less time for daily treatment
- have fewer out-of-pocket treatment expenses

With permission from Augustin M, Radtke MA, Zschocke I, et al. The patient benefit index: a novel approach in patient-defined outcomes measurement for skin diseases. *Arch Dermatol Res.* 2009;301(8):561–571.

Doppler Ultrasonographic Assessment

1. Make the patient comfortable. The patient should be lying flat (if possible for 15–20 minutes before the procedure).
2. Locate the brachial pulse with the Doppler ultrasonograph, apply ultrasound gel and inflate the sphygmomanometer cuff. When the signal fades and disappears, gradually deflate the cuff and record the point at which the signal returns (brachial systolic pressure).
3. Examine the dorsal area of the ulcerated limb and locate the dorsalis pedis pulse (note that this pulse is absent in around 12% of the population). If no pedal pulse can be located, use the posterior tibial pulse. Apply the sphygmomanometer cuff just above the ankle, warning the

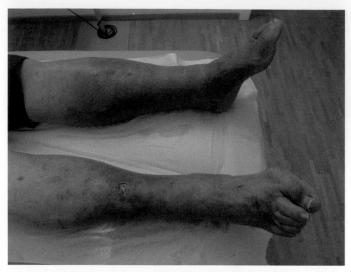

Fig. 9.8 A venous leg ulcer with associated clinical signs.

patient that this procedure may be uncomfortable for a few minutes. Apply ultrasound gel and inflate the cuff, listening carefully for the signal to disappear. Again, gradually deflate the cuff, noting and recording the point at which the signal returns (ankle systolic pressure; Fig. 9.9).

This Doppler assessment is contraindicated in the case of pain or vein thrombosis. Assessment can be made using a manual Doppler or automated equipment.[31] The ABPI must be interpreted with caution. First, the results may be influenced by diabetes or renal disease because these pathologies can result in arterial calcification.[32] Moreover, the results may be influenced by the clinician's skill in taking these Doppler measurements, and so must be performed by an experienced clinician. The results are interpreted as shown in Table 9.4.

Wound Assessment

After assessment of the person and the legs, the LU should be assessed. This examination generally confirms of the wound's aetiology. The localization, form, surface, depth and peripheral skin of the wound reveals the diagnosis.

Tissue viability, infection, moisture and edge (TIME) principles may be used to evaluate and focus on wound bed preparation.

Table 9.1 presents differences in wound and peripheral wound characteristics based on aetiology.

As shown in the epidemiological data, 10% of leg ulcerations can result from vasculitis, malignancy or other disorders. In clinical practice, patients with a non-healing or an atypical leg ulcer must be referred to a specialist for further investigation.[27]

After assessing a person living with an LU, nurses must be able to:

- suggest, if needed, further investigations by a clinical nurse specialist in wound care, doctor or multidisciplinary team member
- implement adequate treatment for the wound based on the patient's needs and wound assessment
- propose person-centred care, including education.

Management

Although a patient with an LU can be assessed in a single session, the wound's management depends partially on its aetiology: venous, arterial or mixed, as well as on some global principles. When reading this section, remember that management of an LU is dynamic and evolving and requires frequent re-evaluation.

GLOBAL MANAGEMENT OF LUS

Evidence-based practice depends on three factors: First, the best evidence in practice, such as literature

TABLE 9.2 Clinical (C) Classes in the CEAP Classification for Chronic Venous Disorders	
Clinical Classification	**Signs**
C0	No visible or palpable signs of venous disease
C1	Telangiectasies or reticular veins
C2	Varicose veins; distinguished from reticular veins by a diameter of 3 mm or more
C3	Oedema
C4	Changes in skin and subcutaneous tissue secondary to chronic venous disorders
C4a	Pigmentation or eczema
C4b	Lipodermatosclerosis or atrophie blanche
C5	Healed venous ulcer
C6	Active venous ulcer
Each clinical class is further characterized by a subscript for the presence of symptoms (S, symptomatic) or absence of symptoms (A, asymptomatic). Symptoms include aching, pain, tightness, skin irritation, heaviness, muscle cramps and other complaints attributable to venous dysfunction	

With permission from Eklöf B, Rutherford RB, Bergan JJ, et al. Revision of the CEAP classification for chronic venous disorders: Consensus statement. *J Vasc Surg.* 2004;40:1248–1252.

reviews or consensus documents, must be used; second, the clinician's competencies must be appropriate; and third, the patient's desires and values are taken into consideration. Guidelines present the best care for the management of LUs, but a global assessment provides perspectives for nursing-specific interventions centred on patients' needs.

Symptom management (pain, odour, etc.) is essential regardless of the aetiology of the LU. Taking into consideration any real-world limitations that may be present, such as a patient's mobility restriction or a patient's treatment costs, allows the nurse to focus on essentials and develop an individual care plan.

TABLE 9.3 Fontaine Classification of Peripheral Arterial Disease	
Stage	**Symptoms**
Stage I	Asymptomatic, incomplete blood vessel obstruction
Stage II	Mild claudication pain in limb
Stage IIA	Claudication at a distance >200 m
Stage IIB	Claudication at a distance <200 m
Stage III	Rest pain, mostly in the feet
Stage IV	Necrosis and/or gangrene of the limb

With permission from Hardman R, Jazaeri O, Yi J, Smith M, Gupta R. Overview of classification systems in peripheral artery disease. *Semin Intervent Radiol.* 2014;31:378–388.

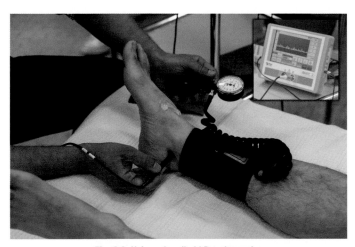

Fig. 9.9 Using a handheld Doppler probe.

Educational intervention should be implemented for each LU aetiology; research has shown that patient understanding of the cause of their LU helps adherence to strategies for healing and reduces recurrence.[33] Patients need to also understand how to promote mobility, avoid trauma on the leg and identify clinical signs or symptoms. Physiotherapy may be recommended for patients who have limited mobility, limited ankle movement or fixed joints. More mobile patients should be encouraged to walk and exercise as much as possible (Figs 9.10 and 9.11). Mobility promotion is important in each kind of LU and depends on the patient's tolerance.

In the case of an LU occurrence, rapid referral to clinical service is important. Elderly patients have a higher risk of developing skin tears, and nurses have to avoid traumatic removal of dressings.

SPECIFIC MANAGEMENT OF VENOUS LEG ULCERS

A VLU is a symptom of the highest grade of venous insufficiency. Compression therapy is the gold standard for reducing recovery time.[34] By improving venous haemodynamics, mechanical compression reduces oedema and improves microcirculation, lymphatic drainage and arterial inflow.[27]

According to Weller et al.[32] there is a lack of clear guidance in relation to the specific ABPI range and safe application of compression therapy. The latest recommendations are presented in Table 9.5. Acute heart failure and arterial occlusive disease are the most important contraindications for compression therapy.

Compression Therapy

Various devices have been developed to apply compression therapy. Examples include elastic, inelastic, multilayer short-stretch or Velcro compression. Fig. 9.12 illustrates one of these devices and Fig. 9.13 illustrates the application of compression bandages. There is no clear evidence to show which is the most effective compression method[34] but research confirms that strong compression (>40 mmHg) improves VLU healing.[27] Recommendations[27] include multicomponent systems or adjustable Velcro devices in the case of untrained professionals.

In practice, nurses must identify two phases, the decongestion phase and the maintenance phase,[35] and adapt devices and frequency of applying bandages

TABLE 9.4 Ankle–Brachial Pressure Index (ABPI) Results and Interpretation	
ABPI	**Perfusion Status**
>1.3	Elevated, incompressible vessels
>1.0	Normal
<0.9	LEAD
<0.6 to 0.8	Borderline
<0.5	Severe ischaemia
<0.4	Critical ischaemia, limb threatened

With permission from WOCN Clinical Practice Wound Subcommittee. Ankle brachial index. *J Wound Ostomy Continence Nurs*. 2012;39(2 Suppl):S21–S9.

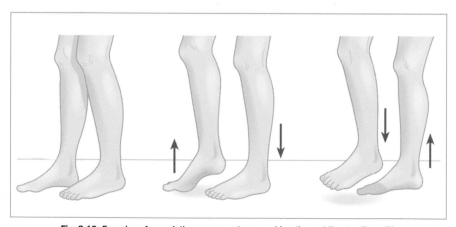

Fig. 9.10 Exercises for assisting venous return: marking time while standing still.

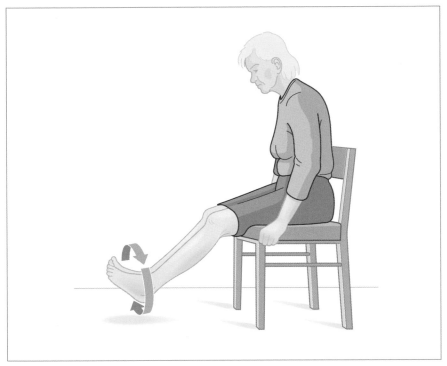

Fig. 9.11 Exercises for assisting venous return: rotate ankles in a circular motion, first one way and then the other.

TABLE 9.5 Ankle–Brachial Pressure Index (ABPI) Results and Guidelines for Applying Compression	
ABPI score	**Intervention**
<0.5	Do not apply compression Referral to specialist is recommended
0.5–0.6	If no rest pain and an absolute pressure above 60 mmHg, graduated compression may be applied by a trained professional Referral to specialist is recommended
0.6–0.8	Graduated compression may be applied by a trained professional Referral to specialist is recommended
0.8–1.2	Apply compression
>1.2	Do not apply compression Referral to specialist is recommended
In slow-healing leg ulcers, the ABPI must be re-assessed every 3 months	

accordingly. The bandages apply two types of pressure on the leg:

- resting: pressure extended when leg is at rest
- working: pressure exerted during muscle work.

Dissemond et al.[35] provide further information on this subject.

To encourage patients to adhere to compression, nurses should initiate compression adequately according to the patient's tolerance. Patients must be informed of symptoms and risk of compression, as they must be able to remove the bandages if needed. During the application of the compression, the clinician must inspect the skin and notice if an inadequate bandage technique does not achieve the right level of compression, as it can have serious implications, such as pressure marks, necrosis or leg ulcer formation.[36] If pain occurs during the compression, the bandages must be removed. Adverse results of compression can be prevented by a complete patient assessment, patient education and clinician experience.[36]

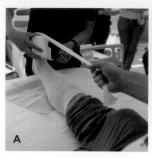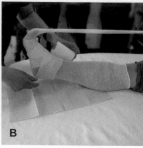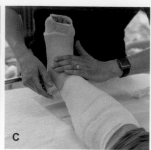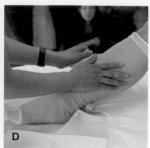

Fig. 9.12 Applying compression bandage needs specific skills. An example of short-stretch bandage with underpadding: (A) tubular gauze and (B) underpadding, (C) first short-stretch bandage, (D) second short-stretch bandage.

Wound Management

Wound management depends on thorough wound bed preparation. It includes as a first step wound cleansing with either a saline solution or tap water, e.g. using a showerhead (according to the law and the quality of running water). Generally, a VLU will present no black necrotic tissue, but yellow slough can occur. A specialized nurse or clinician can remove the devitalized tissue using sharp debridement. If not possible, the devitalized tissue may be removed with appropriate wound cleansing and dressings (e.g., alginate). The wound's edge and surrounding skin have to be protected from moisture to prevent maceration. Generally, the dressing choice will depend on the wound bed, the patient's preferences, the nurse's skills and the available dressings. Because of their high capacity for absorption, hydrofibres, foams and superabsorbent dressings are suitable for an exudative LU. Superabsorbent dressings are preferred because they maintain their humidity-absorbing properties even under compression.

When choosing the dressing, the nurse must remember that the price depends on the material used, but that the selection may also influence the time that will be needed for wound care. As yet, there is no evidence that specific dressings increase the healing rate.[37] The wound healing must be regularly evaluated and the local treatment adapted.

To prevent recurrence in patients with a VLU, compression therapy is required.[27] To improve adherence to treatment, the nurse has to educate the patient, which can be challenging.

Case Study 9.1 explores some issues around taking a holistic approach to VLU management.

SPECIFIC MANAGEMENT OF ARTERIAL LEG ULCERS

The development of ALU is attributed to arterial disease and disrupted blood flow. In this situation, compression is not indicated; it would only reduce the arterial blood flow and promote additional tissue lesions or necrosis. The management of the leg is aimed at re-establishing blood flow if possible. For patients with isolated proximal stenotic or occlusive arterial lesions, percutaneous transluminal angioplasty (PTA) is a useful, minimally invasive procedure. Furthermore, surgery, such as a bypass, can reconstruct the lower limb's arteries by synthetic or autogenous vein grafts, thereby restoring or improving the blood supply (Fig. 9.5B). However, the more distal the damage is, the smaller the artery involved and the more microsurgical techniques using an autogenous graft are preferred. To heal, a wound needs to be vascularized.

During ALU assessment, walking distance and pain evaluation are important to detect arterial obstruction and the need for urgent referral and revascularization. The nursing interventions to the wound will depend on the tissue's viability.

If blood flow does not permit healing, revascularization by percutaneous angioplasty and stent placement or bypass grafting may be proposed and must be discussed by a multidisciplinary team that includes the patient.[25] If no surgical intervention is possible, wound closure will probably not occur. Debridement of necrotic tissue will not be indicated, and wound care should help prevent infection or moisture with use of, for example, polyvinylpyrrolidone iodine (PVP-I) gauze dressings.

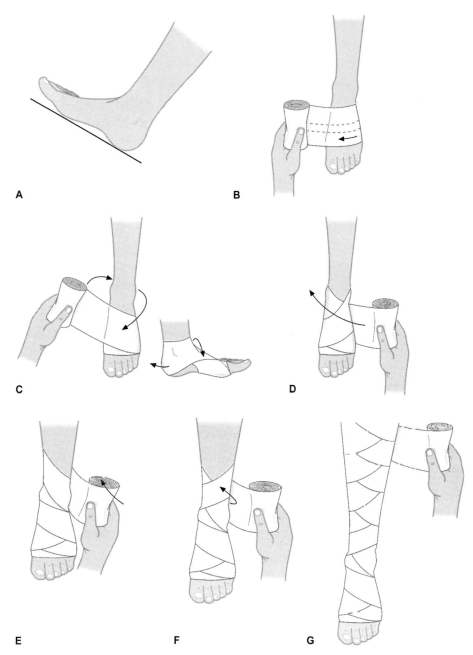

Fig. 9.13 Applying compression bandages in a figure-of-eight. (A) Maintain foot at a right angle to the leg. (B) Make two turns at the base of the toes. (C) Take bandage above the heel. (D) Take bandage around the heel to cover the foot. (E,F) Continue bandaging using figure-of-eight turns. Ensure that 50% stretch is maintained. (G) Bandage up to the tibial tuberosity.

Case Study 9.1

Venous Leg Ulceration

Sara is a 70-year-old woman. She is an active woman who takes care of herself and her grandchildren every weekday. Two months ago, as she walked alongside her grandson on their way home, his bike hurt her leg and caused a small wound. After 2 months of self-care, the wound only grew and became more and more exudative and painful. It reached the point where she had to change her woven compress three times a day, and it regularly spotted her trousers. Because of the pain and shame, she could not walk to the school anymore, nor take care of her grandchildren, which put her daughter in a difficult financial and professional situation.

To correctly assess the situation, the nurse decided to use the theory of goal attainment.[38] During the assessment, the nurse evaluated the three systems from this nursing model (personal, interpersonal, social) and clarified Sara's perception of the situation.

According to the personal system, the nurse acknowledged some risk factors for an LU, including age and sex. She obtained a clear history of the LU and the patient's physical impairments, such as exudation, pain and mobility loss, as well as issues associated with the wound such frequent dressing changes and shame. During physical assessment, the nurse looked for varicosities.

Viewing this case in the light of interpersonal and social systems allowed for identification of the wider issues for Sara, including the wound's effect to limit her role in caring for her grandchildren and the financial repercussions for her daughter. It was important that the nurse understood Sara's perception of the situation. These aspects of Sara's life required a treatment that minimized impairment. In other words, it was important that Sara regained mobility as soon as possible.

According to King,[38] when nurses and clients set mutual goals and agree on modalities, the goal will more likely be attained.

The most important goal for Sara was for the VLU to be healed. The nurse knew this was attainable, but that it would take a long time. Exploring the wider goals together, the nurse and Sara identified the need to improve mobility and avoid dressing leakage so she could return to her role as a grandmother. After their discussion, a care plan was implemented that included physiotherapy, compression bandaging and homecare twice a week for wound care and evaluation.

If further investigation indicates that blood flow permits healing or if the blood flow is re-established, the wound will probably close after wound bed preparation. In this situation, sharp debridement by a trained clinician is recommended.

Pain is a major problem for patients suffering from an ALU. Some treatment plans or advice given by nurses, such as exercising and ambulating, may worsen pain.[25] If no revascularization is possible, pain management will probably require intervention by a multidisciplinary team. With ALUs it is possible to lose part or all of a limb, so a sensitive approach is required.

To have a better outcome regarding wound healing and limb salvaging, patients need to be informed of the negative impact of smoking on arterial disease and wound healing.

SPECIFIC MANAGEMENT OF MIXED LEG ULCERS

Little evidence exists for best practice in MLUs. Identifying an ulceration's major aetiology and the tissue viability are the main indications for treatment approach. Due to its complexity, an MLU must be assessed and managed by a multidisciplinary team. The arterial and venous disease must be investigated completely by an adequate method (e.g., duplex ultrasound). ABPI indicates possible requirement for compression or the need for revascularization. If ABPI is <0.5, no compression must be applied, and the possibility of surgical revascularization must be explored before wound bed preparation. If the APBI is >0.5, modified compression may be implemented while closely monitoring symptoms like pain, appearance of new ulceration or increasing wound size. As well as an ABPI over 0.5, there must be no rest pain for compression to be indicated. The pressure of the bandages must never exceed the arterial perfusion pressure.[36] Some authors[39,40] suggest that with an ABPI above 0.5 and an absolute ankle pressure over 60–70 mmHg, inelastic compression up to 30–40 mmHg may be applied. An ABPI <0.7 may indicate the need for revascularization by bypass or endovascular approach.

Elastic compression maintains a high and constant pressure, which may not be safe in the case of an MLU. In practice, due to the possibility of adverse effects, compression must be initiated with caution and careful supervision.

Case Study 9.2

Mixed Leg Ulceration

Dave is a 68-year-old man who lives alone. He is well known at the outpatient clinic for chronic wounds, where he consults monthly for his venous leg ulceration. Dave has a medical history of hypertension, renal disease and strokes. He also likes to smoke a cigarette with his cup of coffee. This morning, Dave was not expected at the clinic, but he explained that his leg was painful under the compression and that the bandages gave him cramps when he walked. He could not wait for the next week's consultation.

In this case, the nurse used symptom management theory.[41] Through careful history taking, the nurse discovered that Dave had tried some strategies for pain management. He explained that he slept with his right leg hanging off his bed to alleviate the pain. These steps were congruent with the evaluation of his symptoms. However, Dave was not comfortable; he had not found a solution for wearing his compression bandages and did not sleep well. The nurse conducted a physical assessment and observed that Dave's right leg was cold and pale. She performed a Doppler assessment and obtained a ABPI of 0.5. In this case, the nurse reflected on the symptom management strategies and, after discussion with Dave, agreed on the urgent need for a vascular surgeon's evaluation and the potential need for revascularization for symptom management.

Depending on tissue viability, wound bed preparation can be initiated. Wound management will depend on the wound bed evaluation. Most treatments for VLUs or ALUs can be used.

To improve the outcome in mixed aetiologies, patients must be informed of possible complications of arterial disease and encouraged to stop smoking if needed. They must also adhere to treatment and quickly report any adverse effects of compression. Case Study 9.2 explores some of the issues that arise in assessing and managing MLUs.

Conclusion

Patients with LU may need a great deal of psychological support as the effect of chronic ulceration on an individual's quality of life is enormous. Awareness of the problems associated with vascular disease is essential for nurses. Although ulcer healing is the preferred outcome for patients and nurses, in the absence of a real possibility for healing, nurses must focus on the needs and symptoms expressed by their patients.

The key to success in managing patients with LU requires patients' involvement with their treatment. Patients can best take care of themselves, but only if they receive appropriate information and advice, and are truly engaged in their own care. The nurse must remember that many patients will be treated in their own home by the district nurse, or by themselves or caregivers.

FURTHER READING

Atkin L, Bućko Z, Montero EC, et al. Implementing TIMERS: The race against hard-to-heal wounds. *J Wound Care.* 2019;23:S1–S50.

Franks PJ, Barker J, Collier M, et al. Management of patients with venous leg ulcers: challenges and current best practice. *J Wound Care.* 2016;25(Suppl 6):S1–S67.

Greer N, Foman NA, MacDonald R, et al. Advanced wound care therapies for nonhealing diabetic, venous, and arterial ulcers: a systematic review. *Ann Intern Med.* 2013;159(8):532–542.

REFERENCES

1. Nelson EA. Venous leg ulcers. *BMJ Clin Evid.* 2011;2011:1902.
2. Poskitt KR, Gohel MS. Chronic ulceration of the leg. *Surgery (Oxford).* 2016;34:178–182.
3. Graham ID, Harrison MB, Nelson EA, Lorimer K, Fisher A. Prevalence of lower-limb ulceration: a systematic review of prevalence studies. *Adv Skin Wound Care.* 2003;16:305
4. Briggs M, Closs J. The prevalence of leg ulceration: a review of the literature. *EWMA J.* 2003;3(2):14–20.
5. Guest JF, Ayoub N, McIlwraith T, et al. Health economic burden that different wound types impose on the UK's National Health Service: Annual NHS cost of managing different wound types in the UK. *Int Wound J.* 2017;14:322–330.
6. Augustin M, Brocatti LK, Rustenbach SJ, Schäfer I, Herberger K. Cost-of-illness of leg ulcers in the community. *Int Wound J.* 2014;11:283–292.
7. Posnett J, Gottrup F, Lundgren H, Saal G. The resource impact of wounds on health-care providers in Europe. *J Wound Care.* 2009;18. 154–154.
8. Moffatt CJ, Franks PJ, Doherty DC, Smithdale R, Martin R. Sociodemographic factors in chronic leg ulceration. *Br J Dermatol.* 2006;155:307–312.
9. Harrisson MB, Graham ID, Friedberg E, Lorimer K, Vandevelde CS. Assessing the population with leg and foot ulcers. *Can Nurse.* 2001;97:18–23.
10. Persoon A, Heinen MM, van der Vleuten CJM, de Rooij MJ, van de Kerkhof PCM, van Achterberg T. Leg ulcers: a review of their impact on daily life. *J Clin Nurs.* 2004;13:341–354.
11. Moffat C, Vowden P, Téot L. Hard-to-heal wounds: a holistic approach. *EWMA J.* 2008;1–19.

12. Edwards H, Finlayson K, Skerman H, et al. Identification of symptom clusters in patients with chronic venous leg ulcers. *J Pain Symptom Manag*. 2014;47:867–875.
13. Heinen MM, Persoon A, van de Kerkhof P, Otero M, van Achterberg T. Ulcer-related problems and health care needs in patients with venous leg ulceration: a descriptive, cross-sectional study. *Int J Nurs Stud*. 2007;44:1296–1303.
14. Cullum N. *The Nursing Management of Leg Ulcers in the Community: A Critical Review of Research. Report produced for the Department of Health.* Liverpool: University of Liverpool.
15. Burnand KG, Clemenson G, Whimpster I, Browse NL. Proceedings: extravascular fibrin deposition in response to venous hypertension – the cause of venous ulcers. *Br J Surg*. 1976;63(8):660–601.
16. Browse NL. Venous ulceration. *Br Med J Clin Res*. 1983;286(6382):1920–1902.
17. Coleridge Smith PD, Thomas P, Scurr JH, Dormandy JA. Causes of venous ulceration: a new hypothesis. *Br Med J Clin Res*. 1988;296(6638):1726–1727.
18. Fox AD, Budd JS, Horrocks M. Chronic lower limb arterial disease. *Surgery*. 1996:82–88.
19. LeBlanc K, Campbell KE, Wood E, Beeckman D. Best practice recommendations for prevention and management of skin tears in aged skin: an overview. *J Wound Ostomy Cont*. 2018;45:540–542.
20. Blume-Peytavi U, Kottner J, Sterry W, et al. Age-associated skin conditions and diseases: current perspectives and future options. *Gerontol*. 2016;56:S230–242.
21. *International consensus: Optimising wellbeing in people living with a wound.* London: Wounds International; 2012. Available at: https://www.woundsinternational.com/resources/details/international-consensus-optimising-wellbeing-in-people-living-with-a-wound.
22. Moffatt C, Murray S, Keeley V, Aubeeluck A. Non-adherence to treatment of chronic wounds: patient versus professional perspectives. *Int Wound J*. 2017;14:1305–1312.
23. Green J, Jester R, McKinley R, Pooler A. Nurse–patient consultations in primary care: do patients disclose their concerns? *J Wound Care*. 2013;22:534–539.
24. Augustin M, Blome C, Zschocke I, et al. Benefit evaluation in the therapy of chronic wounds from the patients' perspective – development and validation of a new method: patient benefit in chronic wound therapy. *Wound Repair Regen*. 2011;20:8–14. https://onlinelibrary.wiley.com/doi/full/10.1111/j.1524-475X.2011.00751.x.
25. Sieggreen MY, Kline RA. Arterial insufficiency and ulceration: diagnosis and treatment options. *Adv Skin Wound Care*. 2004;17:242–251.
26. Bobbink P, Morin D, Probst S. Evaluation of needs and treatment benefits in outpatient care for leg ulcer patients: a pilot study. *J Wound Care*. 2018;27:527–533.
27. Franks PJ, Barker J, Collier M, et al. Management of patients with venous leg ulcers: challenges and current best practice. *J Wound Care*. 2016;25:S1–S67.
28. Eklöf B, Rutherford RB, Bergan JJ, et al. Revision of the CEAP classification for chronic venous disorders: consensus statement. *J Vasc Surg*. 2004;40:1248–1252.
29. Hardman R, Jazaeri O, Yi J, Smith M, Gupta R. Overview of classification systems in peripheral artery disease. *Semin Intervent Radiol*. 2014;31:378–388.
30. Marin JA, Woo KY. Clinical characteristics of mixed arteriovenous leg ulcers: a descriptive study. *J Wound Ostomy Continence Nurs*. 2017;44:41–47.
31. WOCN Clinical Practice Wound Subcommittee. Ankle Brachial Index. *J Wound Ostomy Continence Nurs*. 2012;39(2 Suppl):S21–S29.
32. Weller CD, Team V, Ivory JD, Crawford K, Gethin G. ABPI reporting and compression recommendations in global clinical practice guidelines on venous leg ulcer management: a scoping review. *Int Wound J*. 2019;16:406–419.
33. Probst S, Allet L, Depeyre J, Colin S, Buehrer Skinner M. A targeted interprofessional educational intervention to address therapeutic adherence of venous leg ulcer persons (TIEIV-LU): study protocol for a randomized controlled trial. *Trials*. 2019;20:243.
34. O'Meara S, Cullum N, Nelson EA, Dumville JC. Compression for venous leg ulcers. *Cochrane Database Syst Rev*. 2012;14(11):CD000265.
35. Dissemond J, Assenheimer B, Bültemann A, et al. Compression therapy in patients with venous leg ulcers. *J Dtsch Dermatol Ges J Ger Soc Dermatol JDDG*. 2016;14(11):1072–1087.
36. Andriessen A, Apelqvist J, Mosti G, Partsch H, Gonska C, Abel M. Compression therapy for venous leg ulcers: risk factors for adverse events and complications, contraindications – a review of present guidelines. *J Eur Acad Dermatol Venereol*. 2017;31:1562–1568.
37. Palfreyman SJ, Nelson EA, Lochiel R, Michaels JA. Dressings for healing venous leg ulcers. *Cochrane Database Syst Rev*. 2014;6(5):CD001103.
38. King IM. *A Theory for Nursing: Systems, Concepts, Process.* New York: Wiley; 1981.
39. Mosti G, Iabichella ML, Partsch H. Compression therapy in mixed ulcers increases venous output and arterial perfusion. *J Vasc Surg*. 2012;55:122–128.
40. Stansal A, Tella E, Yannoutsos A, et al. Supervised short-stretch compression therapy in mixed leg ulcers. *J Med Vasc*. 2018;43(4):225–230.
41. Dodd M, Janson S, Facione N, et al. Advancing the science of symptom management. *J Adv Nurs*. 2001;33:668–676.

MCQS

1 *Which is the most common aetiology of LU?*
a. Venous
b. Arterial
c. Malignancy
d. Mixed

2 *Which of the following is not congruent with arterial disease?*
a. Pale and cold leg
b. Atrophie blanche
c. Necrotic tissue
d. History of hypertension

3 *Which treatment is the gold standard for VLU?*
a. Alginate dressings
b. Hydrocellular dressings
c. Compression ≈40 mmHg
d. Compression 20–30 mmHg

Chapter 10

Cancer and Palliative Wound Care

Sebastian Probst

Highlights

As you read through this chapter, concentrate on the following:

- The importance of the nurse–patient relationship in helping patients understand the nature of their wounds
- The importance of understanding the basic principles of palliative wound management
- Palliative management of a wound when healing is not the outcome
- Psychological aspects

Key Issues

This chapter looks at the challenges of managing cancer-related and palliative wounds. Palliative wound care includes the care of patients, of all ages, with the management of wounds caused by advanced diseases and conditions.

Cancer Wound Care

Case Study 10.1 outlines the case of a woman who has undergone a partial mastectomy for removal of a breast tumour. The suture lines are clean and non-inflamed.

EPIDEMIOLOGY AND AETIOLOGY

Breast cancer is the most common malignancy in women around the world. Information on the incidence and mortality of breast cancer is essential for planning health measures.[1] Breast cancer incidence and death rates generally increase with age.[2] There were about 14.9 million new cases in the world in 2012. It is predicted that this will rise to 22 million new cases per year in two decades.[3]

Risk factors include early menarche, late first pregnancy, late menopause and hereditary influences such as family history of breast cancer. Some risk factors are also related to a women's life stage/hormonal status. For example, one-third of postmenopausal breast cancers are thought to be caused by behavioural factors that are modifiable – postmenopausal obesity, physical inactivity or low activity, use of combined oestrogen and progestin menopausal hormones, alcohol consumption and history of not breastfeeding.[4]

Most breast cancers begin either in the milk-producing glands in breast tissue called lobules, or in the ducts that connect the lobules to the nipple (these arise from the epithelial cells within the terminal duct lobular unit of the breast). The remainder of the breast is made up of fatty, connective and lymphatic tissues.

Breast cancer staging describes the extent to which the cancer has grown and/or spread according to the staging system used:

In Situ Stage

This refers to the presence of abnormal cells that have not invaded nearby tissues (corresponding to stage 0 in the TNM staging system). There are two main types of in situ breast cancer: ductal carcinoma in situ (DCIS) and lobular carcinoma in situ (LCIS), also known as lobular neoplasia. Other in situ breast cancers have characteristics of both ductal and lobular carcinomas or have unknown origins.

Local Stage

This refers to cancers that are confined to the breast (corresponding to stage I and some stage II cancers).

Regional Stage

This refers to tumours that have spread to surrounding tissue or nearby lymph nodes (generally corresponding

Case Study 10.1

*Partial Mastectomy and Breast
Reconstruction*

Mrs Joyce Harris is recovering in hospital following a partial mastectomy and breast reconstruction. The operation
to remove a tumour from her left breast was performed
4 days ago. She now has two transverse suture lines, one
across the reconstructed left breast, the other across her
abdomen from which tissue was taken to perform the
reconstructive surgery.

Joyce, who is 46 years old, is progressing well and is
pleased with the cosmetic results of her breast. She has
been informed that all the tumour was removed but will
require a few weeks of radiotherapy as a precaution.

to stage II or III cancers, depending on size and lymph
node involvement).

Distant Stage

Cancers at this stage are those that have metastasized
(spread) to distant organs or lymph nodes above the
collarbone, they have broken through the walls of the
glands or ducts where they originated and grown into
surrounding breast tissue (corresponding to some
stage IIIc and all stage IV cancers). Most (80%) breast
cancers are invasive or infiltrating.[2]

Although breast cancer is generally referred to as a
single disease, there are up to 21 distinct histological
subtypes and at least four different molecular subtypes
that differ in terms of risk factors, presentation,
response to treatment, and outcomes.[5] Tumour
differentiation can be scored and graded as mentioned
above and this is a useful predictor of the type of
treatment offered, local recurrence and the overall
prognosis for the patient.

Breast cancer is one of the most common cancers
in the world and although its incidence is higher in
some developed countries, death rates are higher in
less developed countries as there is a lower health
literacy level, fewer resources and diagnosis is often
made at a later stage. Therefore, improved screening
and early detection programs in these countries are
needed.[1] As with many chronic conditions, breast
cancer management requires a multidisciplinary
approach, which should include surgery, radiation
and chemotherapy and also genetic expertise, to help

identify genes associated with breast cancer. While
more resources are needed for breast cancer treatment
in general, genetic screening comes at a high cost.
To help ensure early detection and access to care for
all patients, it is important to identify and remove
the socio-economic barriers to accessing healthcare
services that exist.[6]

DIAGNOSIS

Breast cancer is typically detected either during a
screening examination before symptoms have developed, or after a woman notices a lump. Most masses
seen on a mammogram and most breast lumps turn
out to be benign (not cancerous), do not grow uncon-
trollably or spread, and are not life-threatening. When
cancer is suspected, microscopic analysis of breast
tissue is necessary for a diagnosis, to determine the
extent of spread (stage) and to characterize the type of
the disease. The tissue for microscopic analysis can be
obtained from a needle biopsy (fine-needle or wider
core needle) or surgical incision. Selection of the type
of biopsy is based on multiple factors, including the
size and location of the mass, as well as patient factors and preferences, and resources. It is likely that a
number of other investigations will be performed at
this early stage. A full medical history will be taken
by the breast specialist, which is followed by a physical examination including clinical examination of the
breast. Other investigations carried out at this time
may include, as mentioned previously, mammogram,
fine-needle aspiration of the mass or lump for cytol-
ogy (FNAC), ultrasonography to differentiate between
lumps and cysts and magnetic resonance imaging
(MRI). The use of ultrasound instead of mammograms
for breast cancer screening is not recommended; MRIs
should supplement, but not replace, mammography
screening. It will take several days for the results of
these types of investigation to be reported and for the
breast specialist to make a firm diagnosis. This is an
extremely stressful time for the woman and her family.

TREATMENT

A range of treatment options are now available including surgery, radiotherapy, chemotherapy, electrochemotherapy and other adjuvant therapies such as
hormone therapy. The primary goals of breast cancer
surgery are to remove the cancer and determine its

stage. Surgical treatment involves a range of procedures from simple excision of the breast lump (breast-conserving surgery; BCS) to a wide local excision of the lump, partial or segmental mastectomy or simple mastectomy, possibly with axillary dissection of lymph glands. Radiotherapy and/or chemotherapy may be offered in addition to surgery.

POSTOPERATIVE CARE

The suture lines need to be observed for signs of local clinical infection and this observation linked to measurements of body temperature and pulse (as signs of systemic infection). The key elements of postoperative wound care include timely review of the wound, appropriate cleansing and dressing, as well as early recognition and active treatment of wound complications (especially infection and dehiscence). Typically, initial surgical dressings are to remain in place for 48–72 hours and some stay in place for up to 7 days (although not in patients with a higher risk of infection). Around postoperative day 3, the superficial epidermis of a primarily closed incision line may appear 'sealed'. Although the tissue layers are not completely healed and are not able to withstand external forces at this time, the epidermis is the first to resurface, or restratify, to begin to form a barrier to pathogens and contaminants. The primary wound dressing can be left undisturbed if a transparent dressing has been used and only changed if it becomes too soiled. It is also usual for low-suction drainage to be used; one drain is inserted under the suture lines and another in the axillary area, both sites where haematoma formation is likely. After 48 hours, these may be removed when the drainage subsides. The type of drain and need for drainage depends on a range of factors including patient status, grade of tumour, etc.

Nursing Model for Joyce

Joyce requires basic postoperative care for her wounds. The surgery has been elective and at a site with a low risk of contamination. However, think of the wider implications of this type of surgery and the cosmetic and psychological effects this type of wound has on any woman.

Joyce needs to adapt to her new body image and may perceive that she has lost her sexual attractiveness; maybe Roy's adaptation model would be a good choice here (Table 10.1).

Practice Points

- By assessing the focal, contextual or residual origins of the various problems, the nurse can plan appropriate interventions using a person-centred approach.
- What are the major features required to give Joyce optimum care? Wound care may not be the most important issue in this case. The services of the specialist breast nurse should be enlisted to provide support and advice to this patient.

Summary *Key Considerations in Postoperative Wound Care*

- Knowledge of wound healing phases; an understanding of whether a surgical wound is healing by primary, secondary or tertiary intention, and signs of complications
- Topical wound management – types of wound dressings, cleansing solutions and appropriate dressing change regimens.
- Postoperative management of incisional pain.

Careful attention to these aspects of wound care will help to optimize clinical outcomes for postsurgical patients in general.[7,8] Special attention should be given to psychosocial needs in cancer patients.

From Garimella V, Cellini C. Postoperative pain control. *Clin Colon Rectal Surg.* 2013;26(3):191–196; Leaper D, Ousey K. Evidence update on prevention of surgical site infection. *Curr Opin Infect Dis.* 2015;28(2):158–163.

Palliative Wound Care
INTRODUCTION

Palliative care is derived from and associated with the philosophy of the hospice movement. Its purpose is to improve the quality of life for patients and their families facing the problems associated with a life-threatening illness.[9] Improving quality of life requires the appropriate management of symptoms, preventing suffering and providing psychosocial and spiritual support (Fig. 10.1).[10] The literature describes four important attributes of palliative care,[11] which are defined as follows:

TABLE 10.1   Application of Roy's Assessment Model to the Problems of Mrs Harris (Case Study 10.1)

Life Area	Assessment Level 1 – Behaviour	Assessment Level 2 – Stimuli		
		Focal	Contextual	Residual
Physiological: rest and activity	Unable to move arm and sit up straight	Wound painful		Fear of splitting stitches
Physiological: regulation	Pain in breast and abdomen	Surgery, anxiety	Afraid to bother nurses for pain relief	Afraid to take too many painkillers
	Wound dehiscence Wound infection	No obvious signs	Wound breakdown likely at 10 days	
Self-concept	Worried about scarring	Wound sutured	Underlying malignancy may retard healing	Has heard bad reports of breast reconstruction
	Loss of 'normal' body appearance	Left breast shape different from right	Final shape may differ	Breast shape not as shown in pictures of reconstruction
	Fear of recurrence of disease	Only lump removed, not whole breast	Doctors cannot give 100% assurance	Has no experience of others with same problem
Role function	Loss of femininity	Sutured wounds ugly	Feels tired and depressed after operation	
	Loss of role as husband's sexual partner	Husband's anxiety has changed his manner with her		

Total, Active and Individualized Patient Care

This is based on comprehensive symptom management, the goal of which is to reduce suffering and to enhance the physical, emotional, social, spiritual and relational aspect.

Support for the Family

Support for the family is crucial, especially if the disease is advanced. The needs of the patient and family members change over time and at each stage of the palliative care continuum. Examples of the issues identified in palliative care in relation to families include the fear of losing a loved one, anxiety about managing medications and the emotional burden of caring for a terminally ill family member. Palliative care can offer support to patients and their families in this difficult situation and may have a role in helping to reconcile or heal relationships.

Multidisciplinary Team Approach

Fundamental to this model is the provision of multi-professional care based on an interdisciplinary

understanding of a patient's illness covering a breadth of clinical perspectives. This enables a comprehensive and truly person-centred approach to palliative care.[12]

Effective Communication

As part of this interdisciplinary approach, effective communication is important between the patient, family and the healthcare professionals so that advanced care planning can be possible. Good communication about prognosis, care planning and treatment goals is required.

This model provides a useful framework for caring for people with advanced disease symptoms such as malignant fungating wounds.

MANAGEMENT OF PALLIATIVE WOUNDS

Palliative wound care acknowledges the psychosocial impact of the wound on the individual concerned, their social environment such as family and friends, and their clinicians. The following three components contribute to managing such wounds:

- palliation of the underlying cause of the wound
- management of the wound and periwound skin
- management of wound-related symptoms.

These aspects will be illustrated using the example of malignant fungating wounds.

Malignant Fungating Wounds

The psychological problems associated with fungating malignant lesions, as described in Case Study 10.2, can be as great as the physical problems.

Nursing Model for Dorothy

Roy's adaptation model[13] is a useful framework when nursing terminally ill patients. As outlined in Chapter 2, Roy's model is consistent with the hospice philosophy, in that when active treatment is not possible, symptomatic relief will help patients adapt to their particular situation and allow them to come to terms with their illness. Try using this model to plan the care for Dorothy.

AETIOLOGY AND PREVALENCE

A malignant fungating wound is an infiltration of the tumour or the metastasis into the skin and the afferent blood and lymph vessels.[14] Unless the underlying malignant cells are under control, through either chemotherapy, radiotherapy, hormone therapy

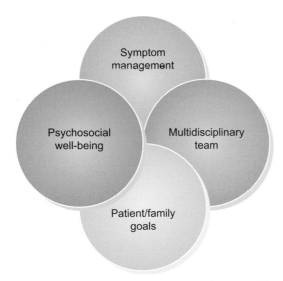

Fig. 10.1 Integrated approach of palliative wound care according to **Emmons and Lachman.** (Emmons KR, Lachman VD. Palliative wound care: a concept analysis. *J Wound Ostomy Continence Nurs.* 2010;37(6):639–644.)

Case Study 10.2

Advanced Breast Cancer and Malignant Fungating Wound (Fig. 10.2)

Mrs Dorothy Brown is a 55-year-old accountant who was admitted to a hospice for management of a fungating carcinoma of her left breast. Although aware of changes in the shape of her breast some 4 years ago, Dorothy chose to ignore it until finally, prompted by her husband, she went to her GP a year ago. By this time she was having discharge from the nipple and the surrounding skin had the characteristic *peau d'orange* (orange peel) appearance. As Dorothy and her worried husband had feared, she had a large tumour underneath her nipple, which had progressed so extensively that surgery was not recommended. Following a short course of chemotherapy and radiotherapy, both Mr and Mrs Brown and her oncologist decided that aggressive treatment was too physically and mentally distressing and that she would prefer palliative treatment only.

On admission to the hospice it was found that the whole area of Dorothy's left breast was covered with fungating, malodorous, sloughy tissue. The malignancy had extended throughout the breast and into the lymphatic system, causing extensive lymphoedema of her left arm and leaving it immobilized.

Dorothy was fairly cheerful, although tired and anxious to return home as soon as possible. She was aware of her prognosis but was reluctant to discuss it openly. She was very distressed by advancing disease so evident in the wound. The odour was upsetting her and she was anxious that something should be done to keep the smell at bay, as she was embarrassed when visitors came to call. While she was at home her husband had, with the district nurse's assistance, been dressing the wound but it now required changing three or four times a day due to the constant leakage of exudate. She was not in any undue pain from the tumour but was becoming increasingly short of breath due to secondary deposits in her lung.

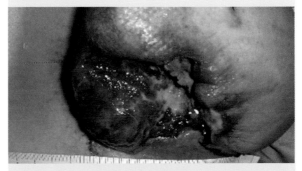

Fig. 10.2 Malignant fungating breast wound.

electrochemotherapy or surgery, the fungation continues growing and consequently the surrounding tissue will be damaged through a combination of loss of vascularity, proliferative growth and ulceration.[15]

It is difficult to determine accurately the number of patients being treated for malignant fungating wounds. There are no exact statistics of malignant fungating wounds across Europe as their incidence rates are not recorded in population-based cancer registers.[14] Most data are based on estimates made within a given population. Lookingbill et al. undertook a retrospective study with 7316 cancer patients looking at the frequency of cutaneous involvement.[16] They reported a rate of 5% of patients with cancer having a malignant fungating wound at diagnosis. In Probst and colleagues' survey, nurses reported a prevalence of malignant fungating wounds of 6.6%. The most frequent area was the breast (49.3%), followed by the neck (20.9%), chest (17.6%), extremities (16.6%), genitalia (16.6%), head (13.5%) and other (1.7%).[17] However, these data were based on self-report rather than prospective data. In summary, it is probable that over 5% of patients with cancer develop a malignant fungating wound. However, with increasing life expectancy with advanced disease and changing cancer therapy this may be increasing.

PSYCHOLOGICAL IMPACT OF THE WOUND

There is only a small amount of research on the psychological impact of malignant fungating wounds on patients and their families. The focus is predominantly on the physical symptoms and daily challenges. Patients often report the unpredictability and uncontrollability of the wound due to symptoms such as malodour, bleeding, exudate and pain. Patients develop strategies to bring the wound symptoms under control. They adopt various methods, often using inadequate products from the medicine cabinet or alternative medicine products. The loss of control of the body boundary due to uncontrollable symptoms lead to significant levels of distress and suffering for patients and their families. Additionally, the visibility of the wound and its visual deterioration provide a constant reminder of having cancer, leading to physical, emotional, psychological and spiritual distress. This results in the loss of sexual identity, fear, anxiety, stress and isolation.[18]

Management

Improvement in the quality of life of patient and family can be achieved by alleviating the distressing symptoms of malodour, bleeding, exudate and pain. It is essential to maintain the patient's dignity and self-esteem by supporting both patient and carers in care of the lesion and adopting a positive outlook to management. Patients may be considered incurable once skin ulceration is present, even without metastases. When treatment with curative intent is no longer appropriate or effective, the focus must shift towards improving quality of life and adopting a positive approach to topical lesion management, as highlighted below.

Local Wound Management

Local wound management is determined by the location, size and shape of the wounds together with presenting problems. However, it must be emphasized that the healthcare professional's attitude, especially during dressing procedures, can greatly influence the patient's own attitude and acceptance of the disease.[19] While physical symptoms can be controlled, the psychological stress of advancing disease can be intensely distressing to patients, carers and relatives.[10]

Management of Wound-Related Symptoms

Symptom management includes both systemic and local aspects. This chapter focuses on the local wound management.

The management of palliative wounds is complex and clinicians managing such wounds need specialist knowledge and expertise in the art and science of symptom control. To achieve this goal, a multidisciplinary approach is needed.

Wound-related symptoms include odour, exudate, spontaneous bleeding, pain, soreness and irritation from excoriated skin. Usually several symptoms have to be taken care of at a given time. The following strategies can help to manage these symptoms:

Clinical Assessment

A clinical assessment of the wound is always required. In the literature, five assessment scales are described: the Toronto Symptom Assessment System for Wounds,[20] the Schulz Malignant Fungating Wound Assessment Tool,[21] the Wound Symptoms Self-Assessment Chart,[22] the TELER System[14,23] and the Hopkins Wound Assessment Tool[24] (Table 10.2). All

TABLE 10.2   Overview of Current Malignant Fungating Wound Assessment Tools

Content	Comments
Toronto Symptom Assessment System for Wounds[a]	
Wound-related symptoms (pain with dressings, pain between dressing changes, exudate/drainage, odour and bleeding) Psychosocial aspects (cosmetic or aesthetic concern, swelling or oedema around the wound, bulk or mass effect from the wound, bulk or mass effect from the dressing)	Retrospective assessment of wound-related symptoms over the previous 24 hours Measurements using a 0–10 visual analogue scale (VAS) Completion either by the patient, with assistance from the caregiver, or by the caregiver
Schulz Malignant Fungating Wound Assessment Tool[b]	
General information about the patient (assessment date, chart number, patient's name, birth date, cancer diagnosis, wound onset date, medical history, medications and allergies) Items concerning the wound (pain with or between dressing changes, location of pain, description of odour and cause, amount of exudate, bleeding – location and quantity, location of oedema, tissue type (in %), wound location, wound dimensions, wound classification (shape of wound), appearance of periwound skin, wound management Items consist of open-ended questions to assess patient's perceptions (How severe? Pain feels like? How much drainage? Do dressings work? Does it affect social activities? How does the wound make you feel? Does it smell? Any swelling?).	Completion by healthcare professionals
Wound Symptoms Self-Assessment Chart[c]	
Wound-related symptoms (pain from the wound, pain during dressing change, leakage of exudate, bleeding from the wound, smell from the wound) Level of interference (mood, anxiety, alertness, attitudes, functional abilities, severity of clinical symptoms)	Completion either by patients or caregivers. Measurement by: (1) a VAS scale (questions on severity of the wound-related symptoms) and (2) a five-point Likert scale (questions on the level of interference)
TELER System[d]	
All aspects of local wound management and psychosocial impact of wounds are covered: discomfort, skin condition from erythematous maceration from exudate, skin stripping from dressings and fixation tapes, periwound irritation, necrotic tissue, sustained dressing fit in order to contain exudate leakage, odour, and intrusion of dressings and dressing changes on day-to-day living	Completion by patients, carers, clinicians The content of a TELER indicator comprises a long-term treatment or management goal (Code 5), negotiated and not imposed on the patient. Each measure is a TELER indicator with six reference points on an ordinal scale The codes of the indicator are written in ordinary language and define six clinically significant steps towards the achievement of the treatment or management goal Indicators are selected for use following the patient and wound assessment. In routine care indicators are only used if the patient has the problem defined by the indicator. In research studies the indicators are selected to answer the research question

Continued

TABLE 10.2 Overview of Current Malignant Fungating Wound Assessment Tools—cont'd	
Content	Comments
Hopkins Wound Assessment Tool[e]	
Wound classifications (wound, predominant colour, hydration, drainage, pain, odour, tunnelling/undermining)	

[a]Maida V, Ennis M, Kuziemsky C. The Toronto Symptom Assessment System for Wounds: a new clinical and research tool. *Adv Skin Wound Care*. 2009;22(10):468–474.

[b]Schulz V, Kozell K, Biondo PD, et al. The malignant wound assessment tool: a validation study using a Delphi approach. *Palliat Med*. 2009;23(3):266–273.

[c]Naylor W. Malignant wounds: aetiology and principles of management. *Nurs Stand*. 2002;16(52):45–53.

[d]Grocott P, Cowley S. The palliative management of fungating malignant wounds – generalizing from multiple-case study data using a system of reasoning. *Int J Nurs Stud*. 2001;38(5):533–545; Grocott P, Blackwell R, Pillay E, Young R. Digital TELER: clinical note-making and patient outcome measures. *Wounds Int*. 2011;2.

[e]Haisfield-Wolfe ME, Baxendale-Cox LM. Staging of malignant cutaneous wounds: a pilot study. *Oncol Nurs Forum*. 1999;26(6):1055–1064.

From Probst S, Grocott P, Graham T, Gethin G. *Recommendations for the Care of Patients with Malignant Fungating Wounds*. London: EONS; 2015. Available from: http://www.cancernurse.eu/documents/EONSMalignantFungatingWounds.pdf

assessment scales evaluate the five 'core' symptoms – odour, pain, exudate, bleeding and itching. Some scales assess psychosocial aspects and impact on daily life. The use of such scales varies widely and there is a lack of evidence to support one over another; clinicians may therefore deem one scale to be more suited to their care setting.

Wound Cleansing

Irrigation is recommended rather than cleaning with a gauze swab. Irrigating with warm (room temperature) saline using a syringe is best.[10]

Swab cultures can sometimes be helpful in determining the need for antimicrobial treatment if the patient shows signs of spreading infection.

Cleansing fungating and ulcerating wounds with antiseptics was originally thought to inhibit bacterial proliferation and diminish the offensive smell of anaerobic infection. Generally, this has been found to be ineffective, as most cleansing agents are inactivated by body fluids.[10] As bleeding points can be easily disturbed, only gentle irrigation with warm water or saline should be undertaken to remove debris and old dressings.

Odour Control

Wound odour can have a profound psychological impact, contributing to stress and negative mood in patients, carers and healthcare professionals. Patients describe wound-related odour as 'rotten' or 'repulsive'.[18] The smell of these tumours is likely to be due to a complex interaction between anaerobic and aerobic organisms.[25] Dead tissue and wound exudate may be contributing factors. The following approaches are commonly used to manage wound-related odour:

- wound cleansing with metronidazole or polyhexanide[26]
- metronidazole (orally or topically) can be helpful[27]
  - metronidazole 500 mg bid or tid orally or intravenously
  - gel or injectable metronidazole can be applied (not injected) on the wound with each dressing change
- application of licenced medical-grade honey
- activated-charcoal and antimicrobial (silver) dressings can help absorb and reduce odour when the dressings completely cover the wounds and contain the volatile substances responsible for the malodour.

Managing wound-related odour in the patient's environment is very challenging. Common actions are over-the-counter room deodorizers, followed by the use of aromatherapy candles and oils.[25] Additional measures are shown in Table 10.3. It has be underlined that the acceptability of these approaches must be discussed with patients and families.

Exudate Management

Malignant fungating wounds have a tendency to produce moderate to high levels of exudate, which results in leakage, soiling, frequent dressing changes, peri-wound maceration and odour. Therefore, an effective exudate control is important. Dressings should fit the margins of the wound precisely to avoid leakage onto clothing and excoriation to the periwound area, and the nurse should find effective methods of fixing the dressing in place. Patients get very distressed when extra padding has to be applied between scheduled dressing changes and when clothes become soiled. Periwound skin (Table 10.4) should be treated with extreme care and the use of barrier skin preparations should be considered.

TABLE 10.3   Strategies for Odour Management in the Environment

Agents	Action
Shaving foam Cat litter Charcoal coals	Odour absorption
Room deodorizers	Room deodorizing
Aromatherapy oils (lavender, bergamot, patchouli, etc.) Dried sage Balsamic vinegar	Odour masking

From Gethin G, Grocott P, Probst S, Clarke E. Current practice in the management of wound odour: an international survey. *Int J Nurs Stud*. 2014;51(6):865–874.

Pain Management

Physical pain is a significant and complex phenomenon in malignant fungating wounds. Pain in palliative wounds may have a nociceptive or/and neuropathic origin. It may be caused by:

- the pressure of the tumour on other body structures
- damage to the nerves caused by the growing tumour
- swelling resulting from impaired capillary and lymphatic drainage
- infections
- exposure of dermal nerve endings
- mismanaged change of wound dressings.

To select the most appropriate treatment and to avoid additional pain during the dressing change an assessment is vital. The following management strategies may be considered:

Topical Application of Morphine and Cannabis

- *Morphine*: Evidence recommends the topical application of opioids. This author considers this to be a safe approach due to the low doses used and the minimal systemic absorption. Dosage varies between 6.25 and 15 mg, with the most common being 10 mg morphine in 8 g hydrogel.[28]

TABLE 10.4   Periwound Management

Type	Description	Application	Comments
Silicone dressings	Inorganic compounds that are insoluble in water Film-forming liquid skin preparation to form a protective interface on skin attachment sites	Apply to still-intact periwound skin (2–3 cm)	Allergy is rare Certain types of silicone products are tacky, facilitating dressing adherence to the skin without any adhesive
Zinc oxide/petrolatum Acrylates	Inorganic compounds that are insoluble in water Film-forming liquid skin preparation to form a protective interface on skin attachment sites	Apply a generous quantity to skin Spray or wipe on still-intact skin surrounding the ulceration (2–3 cm)	May interfere with activity of ionic silver Allergy is uncommon Facilitates visualization of periwound skin
Hydrocolloid or adhesive film dressing	A hydrocolloid wafer consists of a backing with carboxymethylcellulose as the filler, water-absorptive components, such as gelatine and pectin (contained in commercial gelatine desserts), and an adhesive	Window frame the wound margin to prevent recurrent stripping of skin (2–4 cm)	

From Woo KY, Sibbald RG. Local wound care for malignant and palliative wounds. *Adv Skin Wound Care*. 2010;23(9):417–428.

- *Cannabis*: 0.5–1.0 mL cannabis oil (delta-9-tetrahydrocannabinol (THC) 7 mg/mL and cannabidiol (CBD) 9 mg/mL) twice daily directly on the wound and covering with a non-adhesive dressing.[29]

Dressing Changes and Dressings

Dressing changes can be particularly painful. Giving a breakthrough or rescue dose of morphine prior to the dressing change can often be helpful.

Non-adherent or low-adherent dressings should be used. Maintaining the wound in a moist environment will not only reduce dressing adherence but will also protect exposed nerve endings. Most low-adherent dressings can be left on during daily radiotherapy sessions.

A summary of recommended pain management strategies can be found in Table 10.5.

Wound Bleeding/Haemorrhage

Wound bleeding/haemorrhage in malignant fungating wounds occurs because tumour cells erode blood vessels and may be compounded by decreased platelet function within the tumour. This can be distressing for patients, families and healthcare professionals. The following methods can help reduce the incidence of minor bleeds at the dressing changes:

- careful dressing application and removal techniques

TABLE 10.5   Recommendations for Pain Management

Aspect	Recommendations
Prior to the dressing change	Administer an analgesic or booster dose of patient's usual opiate
Analgesic drugs	Refer to the World Health Organization guidelines[a]
Wound cleansing	Irrigation is recommended rather than swabbing
Dressings	Non-adherent and wound dressings moistened with saline
Topical application of opioids	10 mg morphine in 8 g hydrogel[b]
Topical application of cannabis	0.5–1.0 mL cannabis oil[c]

[a]WHO. *Palliative Care*. 2010. Available from: https://www.who.int/cancer/palliative/painladder/en/

[b]Graham T, Grocott P, Probst S, Wanklyn S, Dawson J, Gethin G. How are topical opioids used to manage painful cutaneous lesions in palliative care? A critical review. *Pain*. 2013;154(10):1920–1928.

[c]Maida V, Corban J. Topical medical cannabis: a new treatment for wound pain – three cases of pyoderma gangrenosum. *J Pain Symptom Manage*. 2017;54(5):732–736.

From Probst S, Grocott P, Graham T, Gethin G. *Recommendations for the Care of Patients with Malignant Fungating Wounds*. London: EONS; 2015. Available from: http://www.cancernurse.eu/documents/EONSMalignantFungatingWounds.pdf

TABLE 10.6   Topical Haemostatic Agents

Category	Example	Comments
Natural haemostats	Calcium alginates Collagen Oxidized cellulose	Controls minor bleeds Available as a dressing material Bioabsorbable
Coagulants	Gelatin sponge Thrombin	Risk of embolization
Sclerosing agents	Gelatin sponge Silver nitrate	May cause stinging and burning upon application Leaves a coagulum that can act as a pro-inflammatory stimulus
Fibrinolytic antagonists	Tranexamic acid	Oral agent Gastrointestinal adverse effects (nausea/vomiting)
Astringents	Alum solution Sucralfate	May leave a residue on wound
Vasoconstriction	Adrenaline	Gauze soaked in adrenaline 1:1000 applied with pressure for 10 minutes

From Woo KY, Sibbald RG. Local wound care for malignant and palliative wounds. *Adv Skin Wound Care*. 2010;23(9):417–428.

- maintenance of humidity at the wound/dressing interface
- gentle cleaning techniques.

If bleeding does occur:

- apply direct pressure for 10–15 minutes
- use topical haemostatic agents (Table 10.6)
- radiotherapy can be considered if appropriate for the patient and the tumour is thought to be radiosensitive
- electrochemotherapy can provide a 'vascular lock' and control bleeding.

If a patient is at the end of life and uncontrolled bleeding occurs from a large wound, the use of dark towels/blankets is recommended to mask the blood. This is to decrease anxiety for the patient and family. Sedation with a benzodiazepine is important in this situation.[10]

REFERENCES

1. Ghoncheh M, Pournamdar Z, Salehiniya H. Incidence and mortality and epidemiology of breast cancer in the world. *Asian Pac J Cancer Prev: APJCP.* 2016;17(S3):43–46.
2. American Cancer Society. *Breast Cancer Facts & Figures 2017–2018.* Atlanta: American Cancer Society; 2017.
3. Ferlay J, Soerjomataram I, Dikshit R, et al. Cancer incidence and mortality worldwide: sources, methods and major patterns in GLOBOCAN 2012. *Int J Cancer.* 2015;136(5):E359–E386.
4. Tamimi RM, Spiegelman D, Smith-Warner SA, et al. Population attributable risk of modifiable and nonmodifiable breast cancer risk factors in postmenopausal breast cancer. *Am J Epidemiol.* 2016;184(12):884–893.
5. Dieci MV, Orvieto E, Dominici M, Conte P, Guarneri V. Rare breast cancer subtypes: histological, molecular, and clinical peculiarities. *Oncologist.* 2014;19(8):805–813.
6. Yip CH, Buccimazza I, Hartman M, Deo SV, Cheung PS. Improving outcomes in breast cancer for low and middle income countries. *World J Surg.* 2015;39(3):686–692.
7. Garimella V, Cellini C. Postoperative pain control. *Clin Colon Rectal Surg.* 2013;26(3):191–196.
8. Leaper D, Ousey K. Evidence update on prevention of surgical site infection. *Curr Opin Infect Dis.* 2015;28(2):158–163.
9. WHO. *Palliative Care* 2010. Available from: http://www.who.int/cancer/palliative/en/.
10. Probst S, Grocott P, Graham T, Gethin G. *Recommendations for the Care of Patients with Malignant Fungating Wounds.* London: EONS; 2015. Available from: http://www.cancernurse.eu/documents/EONSMalignantFungatingWounds.pdf.
11. Emmons KR, Lachman VD. Palliative wound care: a concept analysis. *J Wound Ostomy Continence Nurs.* 2010;37(6):639–644; quiz 45-46.
12. Woo KY, Sibbald RG. Local wound care for malignant and palliative wounds. *Adv Skin Wound Care.* 2010;23(9):417–428. quiz 29-30.
13. Roy C, Andrews H. *The Roy adaptation model.* 2nd ed. Stamford, Connecticut: Appleton and Lange; 1999.
14. Grocott P, Cowley S. The palliative management of fungating malignant wounds – generalising from multiple-case study data using a system of reasoning. *Int J Nurs Stud.* 2001;38(5):533–545.
15. Mortimer P. Management of skin problems: medical aspects. In: Doyle D, Hanks G, Cherny N, Calman K, eds. *Oxford Textbook of Palliative Medicine.* 3rd ed. Oxford: Oxford University Press; 2003.
16. Lookingbill D, Spangler N, Sexton F. Skin involvement as the presenting sign of internal carcinoma. A retrospective study of 7316 cancer patients. *Journal of the American Academy of Dermatology.* 1990;22:19–26.
17. Probst S, Arber A, Faithfull S. Malignant fungating wounds – a survey of nurses' clinical practice in Switzerland. *Eur J Oncol Nurs.* 2009;13(4):295–298.
18. Probst S, Arber A, Faithfull S. Malignant fungating wounds: the meaning of living in an unbounded body. *Eur J Oncol Nurs.* 2013;17(1):38–45.
19. Grocott P, Gethin G, Probst S. Malignant wound management in advanced illness: new insights. *Curr Opin Support Palliat Care.* 2013;7(1):101–105.
20. Maida V, Ennis M, Kuziemsky C. The Toronto symptom assessment system for wounds: a new clinical and research tool. *Adv Skin Wound Care.* 2009;22(10):468–474.
21. Schulz V, Kozell K, Biondo PD, et al. The malignant wound assessment tool: a validation study using a Delphi approach. *Palliat Med.* 2009;23(3):266–273.
22. Naylor W. Malignant wounds: aetiology and principles of management. *Nurs Stand.* 2002;16(52):45–53; quiz 4,6.
23. Grocott P, Blackwell R, Pillay E, Young R. Digital TELER: clinical note-making and patient outcome measures. *Wounds Int.* 2011;2.
24. Haisfield-Wolfe ME, Baxendale-Cox LM. Staging of malignant cutaneous wounds: a pilot study. *Oncol Nurs Forum.* 1999;26(6):1055–1064.
25. Gethin G, Grocott P, Probst S, Clarke E. Current practice in the management of wound odour: an international survey. *Int J Nurs Stud.* 2014;51(6):865–874.
26. Villela Castro DL, Santos V, Woo K. Polyhexanide versus metronidazole for odor management in malignant (fungating) wounds: a double-blinded, randomized, clinical trial. *J Wound Ostomy Continence Nurs.* 2018;45(5):413–418.
27. Ramasubbu DA, Smith V, Hayden F, Cronin P. Systemic antibiotics for treating malignant wounds. *Cochrane Database Syst Rev.* 2017;8:CD011609.
28. Graham T, Grocott P, Probst S, Wanklyn S, Dawson J, Gethin G. How are topical opioids used to manage painful cutaneous lesions in palliative care? A critical review. *Pain.* 2013;154(10):1920–1928.
29. Maida V, Corban J. Topical medical cannabis: a new treatment for wound pain-three cases of pyoderma gangrenosum. *J Pain Symptom Manage.* 2017;54(5):732–736.

MCQS

1 *During an assessment of a patient with primarily closed surgical incision on postoperative day 5, which of the following could represent development of a surgical site infection?*
a. Erythema of wound margins
b. Increasing exudate
c. Periwound oedema
d. A six out of ten pain rating

2 *Utilizing non-adherent dressings and warming the wound cleansing solution are strategies intended to:*
a. Decrease risk for surgical site infection
b. Decrease risk for wound dehiscence
c. Reduce incision healing time
d. Reduce surgical incision-related pain

3 *Dressings applied to primarily closed surgical incisions should:*
a. Contain topical antibiotics
b. Apply pressure to the incision line
c. Act as a barrier to trauma
d. Repel exudate

4 *Which of the following is a typical duration for an initial surgical wound dressing?*
a. 12–24 hours
b. Less than 12 hours
c. 24–28 hours
d. 48–72 hours

EVALUATION

Chapter 11

Ways of Evaluating Care

Sinéad Hahessy

Key Issues

Evaluation as a a concept is discussed by focusing on four key areas in this chapter
- Evaluation of the wound
- Evaluation of care delivery
- Evaluation of the patient
- Evaluation role of the specialist nurse

Introduction

Today's healthcare practice operates in an ever-changing global culture and has adopted the managerial principles espoused by corporate governance. Issues such as accountability, risk assessment, patient safety and maintaining quality are key in determining the contours of clinical practice. Furthermore, media reports and public pressure have helped identify areas in healthcare that are falling short and putting patients at risk. Necessary healthcare reforms have seen the old approach of trial and error meet its demise in relation to wound management, and evidence-based practice now informs it. Government directives have also defined professional competencies and practice frameworks out of a need to raise standards in this area.

Evaluation and risk assessment is the initial component of clinical decision making and is central to appropriate wound care management. Developing an aptitude for effective and accurate evaluation is key to working with patients with wounds.

Evaluation of the Wound

Evaluation of a wound should commence with observation of shape, colour and the status of the surrounding skin. This is then followed by wound measurement; the same method should be used each time with the patient in the same position. Measuring the wound can indicate whether the wound is improving, deteriorating or static.[1-4] A good indicator of healing is a 30% or more change in the surface area of the wound over a 4-week period. The techniques used in wound measurement can vary from simple length measurement, ideally using a paper ruler, to more technological computer-based and/or digital photography methods, for example histogram planimetry (HP) or Visitrak. Wound measurement using imaging software saves time and is particularly helpful for accurately measuring uneven or jagged-edged wounds.

Measuring the depth of the wound is also important. Wound depth is a measurement of the deepest part of the visible wound bed. In unstageable wounds where necrotic tissue is close to the skin surface, visualization of the true depth of the wound is not possible. Morgan[5] advocates using a sterile cotton tip swab, which is gently inserted into the area and then measured against a ruler. The cavity should be investigated by gently probing and the deepest part of the wound is recorded. Using liquid (sterile saline) is also recommended to determine the fill capacity of the hollow part of the wound. Clear and accurate records should be completed in a timely manner after evaluating a wound and documents should identify risks and plans to address any risk.

Evaluating Delivery of Care

Evaluation of the delivery of healthcare emerged in the wave of a global focus on clinical governance and is now an integral part of contemporary healthcare culture and practice. Concurrently, the growing interest of service users in healthcare-related quality issues has informed governance frameworks that primarily focus on improving patient outcomes. The emergence of 'patient advocacy', 'patient empowerment' and 'accountability' has likely preceded this public interest in healthcare; the era of the patient as a passive recipient of care has passed. Patient empowerment is a personal and political process which alters the power differential between healthcare provider and recipient. In the daily care of patients, this can be challenging in terms of who holds the power and how the clinician–patient relationship is negotiated. The broad aim of patient empowerment is to enable patients to assume more control over their illness and care trajectory.[6] However, 'empowerment' can have different interpretations depending on the patient cohort. Selman et al.[7] found that 'self identity' emerges as a prominent theme for patients with life-limiting conditions, while Richardson et al.[8] found that staying connected to 'a modicum of autonomy' in daily decisions about care empowers patients. The movement towards patient involvement in their own care has now extended to the inclusion of patients and their views in the development of clinical guideline, as discussed by van der Weijedin et al.[9] The Internet has also facilitated the emergence of a more informed public, adding further impetus to ensuring healthcare professionals are accountable and transparent.

Clinical governance is the framework for ensuring best possible patient outcomes, ensuring patient safety and optimizing the quality of healthcare. It is based on a set of related concepts: risk assessment and management, clinical effectiveness, patient experiences, communication, strategic effectiveness, resource effectiveness and learning and staff development. This group of interlinked concepts functions to capture the complexity of healthcare encounters across a range of diverse environments. The concepts do not operate in isolation but exist in a mutually dependent relationship depending on the healthcare context and clinical focus of care. The evaluation of care takes place against this clinical and socio-political backdrop. To ensure clinical effectiveness of a given treatment plan, the evaluation of care should be done through the process of clinical audit.

CLINICAL AUDIT AND NURSING METRICS

Clinical audit is a process that measures the quality of care and is usually conducted by doctors and nurses. In an audit, performance can be measured against a standard and opportunities to improve are identified. Changes in practice can ensue and the audit cycle can continue through the use of further audits to measure if the change was successful. The data generated are used as evidence that the change was, or was not, beneficial. Clinical audit is conducted in a spirit of enhancing the quality of care delivery and is related to clinical effectiveness. Ideally the audit should be a multidisciplinary practice which is directed by the clinical leadership team with strategic aims. Audits can be retrospective or prospective and are usually linked to standard setting. Standard setting aims to provide a level of systematization to clinical care. The systematic approach to clinical practice has been identified by Degeling et al.[10] as a means of making clinical governance function effectively.

The adoption of corporate principles in the management and reform of the healthcare sector has directed clinicians' attention toward the importance of evidenced-based care. The ability to utilize the best available evidence has required nurses to develop the ability to discern what kinds of evidence are valid and appropriate for nursing practice. Developing competency in reviewing evidence is important and can be maintained by continuing professional education which is linked to clinical governance goals. Evidenced-based care has become a key indicator in determining the quality of healthcare practice. Over the past 20 years, the American Nurses Association has been compiling nursing metrics and quality indicators in The National Database of Nursing Quality Indicators (NDNQI),[11] providing valuable information about patient cohorts in the USA. The benefits of using nursing metrics range from provision of real-time data and information to enhancing staff engagement, clinical leadership and accountability. The data produced by clinical audit and nursing metrics can be used in conjunction with other evidence from the literature and research to aid the development of appropriate clinical guidelines.

CLINICAL GUIDELINES

Clinical guidelines are defined as a set of criteria or principles that guide action, and the development of guidelines is underpinned by using the best available evidence. The evidence is used in conjunction with patient values, clinical expertise, economic cost and local need. The development of guidelines in wound care should aim to guide the practitioner to make an appropriate choice of wound dressing.

The advantages of guidelines include the following:
- promote evidence-based practice
- reduce variation in practice and service delivery
- avoid unnecessary duplication
- facilitate effective staff induction
- act as an educational tool
- act as a basis for audit, evaluation and continuous improvement
- meet National Institute for Healthcare Excellence (NICE) standards and local standards
- promote clear governance in the development and implementation of policy, protocol and guidelines.

Regardless of how robust a guideline is, a degree of clinical decision making should be employed in interpreting and applying knowledge. Practitioners should assess the applicability of guidelines to a particular clinical situation by taking into account local circumstances and the needs and wishes of individual patients.

IMPORTANCE OF CLINICAL GOVERNANCE AND NATIONAL STANDARDS

During the 1990s, while the use of clinical governance as a framework for safe practice was being adopted, the media was reporting failures in the health services ranging from inconsistencies in care to more sinister outcomes. The most notable of these relates to the Bristol Royal Infirmary Inquiry (2001), in which investigations of 23 deaths of paediatric patients revealed unacceptable variations in clinical practices. Other cases that came to light were: The Royal Liverpool Children's Inquiry (Alder Hey Inquiry), the case of the GP Harold Shipman and the trial of the nurse Beverly Allitt in 1993. As mentioned previously, clinical governance aims to address failings and promote a systematic approach to care by guiding practice through the development and use of standards, policy and guidelines.

NATIONAL STANDARDS IN WOUND CARE

The Commissioning for Quality and Innovation (CQUIN) has listed wound assessment as one of its targets. The adoption of a systematic approach to wound care at a national level can only occur if communication between practitioners is improved to reduce inconsistencies in care.[12] Using standards can help develop a common language and foster a culture of continuity when evaluating wound care.

WHY SET STANDARDS?

Clinical standards can specify what is to be measured and used as a means of evaluating the level of care given. Standards that directly affect the level of care given are concerned with knowledge (evidence) and skills (competency). Written standards allow practice to be critically examined. It is a way of bridging the theory/practice gap and highlights where resources, knowledge and skills need enhancing to improve practice and patient outcomes. Standard setting gives nurses and other professionals an opportunity to identify what they are trying to achieve and discover whether they achieve it. Traditionally, evaluation of medical and nursing intervention has been primarily focused on quantitative measurement; however the move toward holistic models of care has emphasized the need to address the subjective realm of the patient experience by capturing qualitative data. In wound care, the patient's quality of life has emerged as an important area of research.

Evaluating the Patient's Quality of Life

When evaluation of a wound shows that skin integrity has been achieved, an emotional process has also taken place that is more often ignored. It is difficult to quantify the emotional aspects experienced by patients. However, qualitative data from the subjective perspective of the patient reveals the considerable psychosocial challenges related to living with a wound, and consideration should be given to the this aspect of patient care.

The patient's quality of life will vary between individuals depending on social and educational status, social support and the presence of comorbid factors. It can be argued that nurses will have already identified these as important aspects of a patient's overall care, given that most nursing models address these core areas in their assessment framework. Quality of life (QoL) questionnaires (primarily psychometric) can be used to enhance the evaluation of these aspects of patient experience. Patients with chronic wounds have reported feeling that they have a sense of losing control, have psychological issues related to body image, depending on the kind of wound they have, and may have issues with wound odour and appearance, which can have a deleterious effect on a patient's mood, coping ability and self-concept. For some, wound pain can lead to disruption in sleep patterns and limitations with regards to mobility, all of which will have an effect on quality of life. Depressive symptoms and anxiety are not uncommon in patients with chronic wounds.[13–15]

There are a range of QoL assessment tools available, as comprehensively outlined by Renner and Erfurt-Berge.[16] The Freiburg Life Quality Assessment for wound patients (FLQA-w) includes questions related to physical ailments, everyday life, social life, psychological wellbeing, therapy and satisfaction. The FLQA-w was tested for validity by Augustin et al.[17] and was found to be a reliable assessment tool. The Wound-QoL is a shortened combination (17 of 92 questions) of the FLQA-w, the Cardiff Wound Impact Schedule and the Würzburg Wound Score. The Wound-QoL has three subscales, including everyday life, body and psyche. The Dermatology Quality of Life Index (DLQI) is a 10-item questionnaire that focuses on six areas: symptoms and feelings, daily activities, leisure, work and school, personal relationships, and treatment. The DLQI can be used for over 33 different dermatological diseases and is available in 32 countries and in 55 languages. The EuroQol-5D (EQ-5D) assesses five aspects of life: mobility, self-care, daily activities, pain and anxiety/depression, and includes a scale of 0 to 100 for the patient's health status.

Evaluating the Contribution of the Specialist Nurse

Finally, it is appropriate to review the role of specialist nurse and evaluate the unique skill set that can influence overall care management and the quality of patient care. The clinical nurse specialist is now a well-established part of the NHS whose contribution has clearly influenced the type of care patients with wounds can expect to receive. Although the role developed in North America in the 1960s, it was not until the beginning of 1980 that posts were created in the UK. Specialist and advanced nursing practice roles continue to evolve globally.[18]

Hutchinson et al.[19] have argued that the domains central to the role of the advanced nurse practitioner are autonomous practice; improving systems of care; improving practice development; contributing to education, research and scholarship; and clinical leadership. It could be argued that these domains of practice are mirrored in the principles espoused by clinical governance frameworks. Specialist and advanced nursing practice requires the nurse to recognize the importance of the transition to specialist/advanced practice and to reflect on his/her current role while developing specialist/advanced roles, especially in the early stages. These domains of advanced practice as outlined by Hutchinson et al.[19] can help create a tentative framework for the development of the specialist/advanced practice role and at the same time focus on core areas that contribute to the enhancement of patient care.

BENEFITS OF SPECIALIST AND ADVANCED NURSING

McConkey and Hahessy[18] have explored the application of two domains of practice: autonomous practice and improving systems of care.

In terms of autonomous practice, the advanced nurse practitioner needs to develop the skill of clinical decision making by recognizing the competing paradigms that underpin it. The hypothetico-deductive or scientific approach is based on information processing and is rooted in the biomedical model of healthcare. The intuitive-humanist model places attention on the knowledge that is accumulated from professional experience and intuition.[20] These paradigms speak to the art and science of nursing practice and their influence, interrelationship and sometimes opposition are often overlooked when considering our worldview of nursing. Making appropriate clinical decisions when evaluating wounds requires that a nurse develops competency with experience. This can be supported and sustained by ongoing professional development and education.

Specialist and advanced nurse practitioners have the potential to improve systems of care and this places the nurse at the forefront of clinical leadership. However this aspect of the role requires multidisciplinary support from key stakeholders to be effective. A culture of change management helps to ensure consistency in delivering standards of care through service audits and constant re-evaluation, and this becomes central to the role of the advanced nurse practitioner in wound care. Further research on the benefits and challenges of advanced nursing practice in the area of wound care is required to develop a professional development framework for the role.

Practice Point

If you work with wound care specialists, think of ways in which they improve the quality of care the patient receives.

Summary

Evaluation of care can be achieved in many different ways. Each method concentrates on a particular aspect of wound care. Evaluation should always be considered at the assessment and planning phase of management, not as an afterthought.

The main areas of evaluation can be summarized as follows:

EVALUATION OF THE WOUND
- Wound measurement techniques

EVALUATION OF THE DELIVERY OF CARE
- Clinical audit and nursing metrics
- Guidelines
- Standard setting

EVALUATION OF THE PATIENT
- Quality of life

EVALUATION OF THE NURSE
- Role of the specialist and advanced practitioner nurse in wound care

REFERENCES

1. Margolis D, Allen-Taylor L, Hoffstad O, et al. The accuracy of venous leg ulcer prognostic models in a wound care system. *Wound Repair Regen.* 2004;12:163–168.
2. Rivolo M. Clinical innovation: SEE & WRITE – a new approach for effective recording. *Wounds Int.* 2015;6(2):6–10.
3. Sheehan P, Jones P, Caselli A, Giurini J, Veves A. Percent change in wound area of diabetic foot ulcers over a 4-week period is a robust predictor of complete healing in a 12-week prospective trial. *Diabetes Care.* 2003;26(6):1879–1882.
4. Kantor J, Margolis DJ. A multicentre study of percentage change in venous leg ulcer area as a prognostic index of healing at 24 weeks. *Br J Dermatol.* 2000;142(5):960–964.
5. Morgan N. Measuring wounds. Wound Care Advisor.2012. Available at http://woundcareadvisor.com/measuring-wounds.
6. Barr PJ, Scholl I, Bravo P, Faber MJ, Elwyn G, McAllister M. Assessment of patient empowerment – a systematic review of measures. *PloS One.* 2015;10(5):e0126553.
7. Selman LE, Daveson BA, Smith M. How empowering is hospital care for older people with advanced disease? Barriers and facilitators from a cross-national ethnography in England, Ireland and the USA. *Age Ageing.* 2016;46(2):300–309.
8. Richardson K, MacLeod R, Kent B. Ever decreasing circles: terminal illness, empowerment and decision-making. *J Prim Health Care.* 2010;2(2):130–135.
9. Van der Weijden T, Pieterse AH, Koelewijn-van Loon MS, et al. How can clinical practice guidelines be adapted to facilitate shared decision making? A qualitative key-informant study. *BMJ Quality Safety.* 2013;22(10):855–863.
10. Degeling PJ, Maxwell S, Iedema R, Hunter DJ. Making clinical governance work. *BMJ.* 2004;329(7467):679–681.
11. American Nurses Association. *The National Database of Nursing Quality Indicators (NDNQI)*; 2011. Available from: http://www.nursingworld.org.
12. Vowden P, Vowden K. Clinical care implications of the 'Burden of Wounds' study. *Wounds UK.* 2016;12(3):12–21.
13. Mapplebeck L. Case study: psychosocial aspects of chronic bilateral venous leg ulcers. *Br J Commun Nurs.* 2008;13:33–38.
14. Ousey K, Edward KL. Exploring resilience when living with a wound – an integrative literature review. *Healthcare (Basel).* 2014;2(3):346–355.
15. Zhou K, Jia P. Depressive symptoms in patients with wounds: a cross-sectional study. *Wound Repair Regen.* 2016;24(6):1059–1065.
16. Renner R, Erfurt-Berge C. Depression and quality of life in patients with chronic wounds: ways to measure their influence and their effect on daily life. *Chronic Wound Care Management and Research.* 2017;4:143–151.
17. Augustin M, Herberger K, Rustenbach SJ, Schäfer I, Zschocke I, Blome C. Quality of life evaluation in wounds: validation of the Freiburg Life Quality Assessment-wound module, a disease-specific instrument. *International Wound Journal.* 2010;7(6):493–501.
18. McConkey R, Hahessy S. Developing the advanced nursing practice role in non-muscle invasive bladder cancer surveillance in Ireland. *Int J Urol Nurs.* 2018;12:91–95.
19. Hutchinson M, East L, Stasa H, Jackson D. Deriving consensus on the characteristics of advanced practice nursing: meta-summary of more than 2 decades of research. *Nurs Res.* 2014;63(2):116–128.
20. Nyatanga B, Vocht HD. Intuition in clinical decision-making: a psycho-logical penumbra. *Int J Palliat Nurs.* 2008;14(10). 492–433.

MCQS

1 *What is clinical governance?*
   a. It is a framework for change
   b. It is a nursing model
   c. It is a professional development model
   d. It is a process for governing clinical practice to ensure safety and quality in the delivery of healthcare

2 *Visitrak is:*
   a. A wound dressing
   b. A model of care
   c. A philosophical approach
   d. A computer-based software programme to measure wound depth

3 *A clinical audit is:*
   a. An approach to nursing care
   b. A clinical guideline
   c. A nursing framework
   d. A process to measure the clinical effectiveness of an aspect of clinical practice

Glossary

Abscess: A collection of pus, which has localized. It is formed by the liquefactive disintegration of tissue and a large accumulation of polymorphonuclear leucocytes

Albumin: A water-soluble protein. Serum albumin is the chief protein of blood plasma. It is formed principally in the liver and makes up about four-sevenths of the 6–8% protein concentration in plasma

Alginates: A group of wound dressings derived from seaweed

Anaerobic bacteria: Bacteria that thrive in an oxygen-free environment

Angiogenesis: The process of new blood vessel formation

Antibiotic: A chemical substance that is able to kill or inhibit the growth of micro-organisms. Antibiotics are classified according to their action on the micro-organism

Arteriosclerosis: A group of diseases characterized by thickening and loss of the elasticity of the arterial walls

Aseptic technique: A method of carrying out sterile procedures so that there is the minimum risk of introducing infection. This is achieved by the use of sterile equipment and a non-touch method

Autolysis: The breakdown of devitalized tissues. The disintegration of cells or tissues by endogenous enzymes

Bacteria: Any prokaryotic organism. These are single-celled micro-organisms that lack a true nucleus and organelles. A single loop of double-stranded DNA makes up their genetic material

Callus: Localized hyperplasia of the horny layer of the epidermis caused by friction or pressure

Cauterization: The application of heat sufficient to scar tissue; used to obtain haemostasis

Cellulitis: Inflammation of the subcutaneous tissues. It is characterized by oedema, redness, pain and loss of function

Collagen: The main protein constituent of white fibrous tissue (skin, bone, tendon, cartilage and connective tissue). It is composed of bundles of tropocollagen molecules, which contain three intertwined polypeptide chains

Colonization: The presence of commensal or pathogenic organisms that multiply on the wound but do not cause infection

Contractures: Abnormal shortening of muscle or scar tissue rendering the muscle highly resistant to stretching. A contracture can lead to permanent disability

Debridement: The removal of foreign matter or devitalized, injured, infected tissue from a wound until the surrounding healthy tissue is exposed

Dehiscence: A splitting open or separation of the layers of a surgically closed wound

Devitalized: Devoid of vitality or life; dead

Doppler ultrasonography: A method of measuring blood flow in peripheral arteries. Changes in blood flow may be correlated with pressure gradients across stenosed vessels and valves and can give an indication of blood supply to the distal tissues

Endothelium: The layer of epithelial cells that line the cavities of the heart and of the blood and lymph vessels and of the serous cavities of the body

Epithelialization: The growth of epithelium over a denuded wound surface

Eschar: Dead, devitalized tissue

Extravasation: A discharge or escape of blood or fluid from a vessel in the tissues. Commonly associated with intravenous infusions

Exudate: Wound fluid with a high content of protein and cells that has escaped from blood vessels

Fibroblast: An immature collagen-producing cell of connective tissue

Foam dressing: A dressing material which consists of polyurethane

Fungate: To produce fungus-like growths; to grow rapidly

Granulation tissue: The new tissue formed during the proliferative phase of wound healing. It consists of connective tissue cells and ingrowing young vessels, which form a cicatrix

Haematoma: A localized collection of blood which can form in an organ, space or tissue

Haemostasis: The process of stopping bleeding, which can occur naturally by clot formation or artificially by compression or suturing

Hydrocolloid: A dressing material made up of a colloid in which water is the dispersion medium

Hydrofibre: An absorbent dressing material that transforms into a gel on contact with wound fluid

Hydrogel: A dressing material which consists of a water-containing gel

Hypergranulation/overgranulation: Exuberant amounts of soft, oedematous granulation tissue developing during healing

Hypertrophic: An increase in volume of tissue produced by enlargement of existing cells

Incidence: The proportion of a defined group of patients developing a medical condition in a defined period of time

Infection: The invasion and multiplication of micro-organisms in body fluids or tissues. The spectrum of infection agents continually changes as bacteria and viruses are capable of rapid mutation

Inflammation: The initial response to tissue injury. The inflammatory response can be caused by physical, chemical and biological agents

Ischaemia: The deficiency in blood supply to a part of the body due to functional constriction or actual obstruction of a blood vessel

Keloid: A type of scar, which is often red and prominent. It is caused by excessive collagen formation in the dermis during connective tissue repair

Keratin: An insoluble protein forming the principal component of epidermis, hair, nails and tooth enamel

Leucocyte: Colourless blood corpuscle whose chief function is to protect the body against micro-organisms

Lymphocyte: Mononuclear, non-granular leucocyte, chiefly a product of lymphoid tissue, which participates in the immune response

Maceration: Excessive moisture and redness in the tissues surrounding a wound edge

Macrophage: Any of the large, mononuclear, phagocytic cells derived from monocytes that are found in the walls of blood vessels and in loose connective tissue. They become stimulated by inflammation on initial angiogenesis

Matrix: The intracellular substance of a tissue which forms the framework of tissues

Maturation: A phase in wound healing where scar tissue is remodelled

Myofibroblast: A differentiated fibroblast containing the ultrastructural features of a fibroblast and a smooth muscle cell, and containing many actin-rich microfilaments

Necrosis: The death of previously viable tissue

Prevalence: The proportion of a defined group of patients who have a medical condition at a given time

Proliferation: The growth or reproduction of tissue as part of the healing process

Proline: A cyclic amino acid occurring in proteins; it is a major constituent of collagen

Pus: A protein-rich liquid that consists of exudate, dead macrophages and bacteria

Scab: The dry crust forming over an open wound, which consists of skin and debris

Septicaemia: Blood poisoning, a systemic disease where pathogenic micro-organisms are present and multiply in the blood. It is a life-threatening disease

Slough: A mass of dead tissue in or cast out of living tissue

Superabsorbent dressing: A multilayer wound cover, which combines a semi- or non-adherent layer with highly absorptive layers

Suppuration: Formation of discharge or pus

Suture: A stitch or series of stitches made to secure opposition of the edges of a surgical or traumatic wound

Useful Websites

(This list does not aim to be comprehensive)

American Board of Wound Healing (ABWH): https://abwh.net/

American Association of Diabetes Educators: https://www.diabeteseducator.org/

American Burn Association: http://ameriburn.org/

American Diabetes Association: http://www.diabetes.org/

American Society of Plastic Surgeons: https://www.plasticsurgery.org/

Association for the Advancement of Wound Care: https://aawconline.memberclicks.net/

Cochrane Library: https://www.cochranelibrary.com/ (subscription only)

Debra International: http://www.debra-international.org/

European Council of Enterostomal Therapy: https://ecet-stomacare.eu/

European Pressure Ulcer Advisory Panel (EPUAP): http://www.epuap.org/

European Tissue Repair Society (ETRS): https://www.ctrs.org/

European Wound Management Association (EWMA): http://ewma.org/

International Lymphoedema Framework: https://www.lympho.org/

International Skin Tear Advisory Panel (ISTAP): http://www.skintears.org/

International Wound Infection Institute: http://www.woundinfection-institute.com/

National Institute for Clinical Excellence (NICE): https://www.nice.org.uk/

National Pressure Injury Advisory Panel (NPIAP) https://npiap.com

New Zealand Wound Care Society: https://www.nzwcs.org.nz/

NHS Centre for Reviews and Dissemination: https://www.york.ac.uk/crd/

Nursing and Midwifery Council: https://www.nmc.org.uk/

Royal College of Nursing (RCN): https://www.rcn.org.uk/

Society for Vascular Surgery (SVS): https://vascular.org/

Tissue Viability Society (TVS): https://tvs.org.uk/

World Alliance for Wound & Lymphedema Care (WAWLC): https://wawlc.org/

World Union of Wound Healing Societies: https://www.wuwhs.com/web/

World Wide Wounds: http://www.worldwide-wounds.com/

Wound Information Network: https://webcme.net/win/

Wound Care Society: www.woundcaresociety.org

Wound Healing Society: https://woundheal.org/

Wounds Australia: https://www.woundsaustralia.com.au/

Wounds Canada: https://www.woundscanada.ca/

Answers to MCQs

Chapter 1

1. (c)
2. (b)
3. (d)

Chapter 2

1. (d)
2. (a)
3. (d)

Chapter 3

1. (c)
2. (d)
3. (a)

Chapter 4

1. (c)
2. (d)
3. (c)

Chapter 5

1. (a)
2. (d)
3. (b)

Chapter 6

1. (c)
2. (c)
3. (a)

Chapter 7

1. (a)
2. (b)
3. (c)
4. (a)

Chapter 8

1. (c)
2. (c)
3. (a)

Chapter 9

1. (a)
2. (b)
3. (c)

Chapter 10

1. (a)
2. (d)
3. (c)
4 (d)

Chapter 11

1. (d)
2. (d)
3. (d)

Index

Note: Page numbers followed by "f" indicate figures, "t" indicate tables, and "b" indicate boxes.